AF341991

AUTONOMIC NERVOUS SYSTEM (ANS)

CLINICAL FEATURES, FUNCTIONS AND DISORDERS

HUMAN ANATOMY AND PHYSIOLOGY

Additional books in this series can be found on Nova's website
under the Series tab.

Additional e-books in this series can be found on Nova's website
under the eBooks tab.

AUTONOMIC NERVOUS SYSTEM (ANS)

CLINICAL FEATURES, FUNCTIONS AND DISORDERS

PATRICK BERNARD OWENS
EDITOR

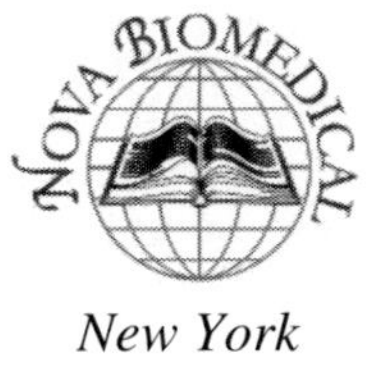

New York

NOTICE TO THE READER

Library of Congress Cataloging-in-Publication Data

ISBN: 978-1-63484-884-8

Library of Congress Control Number: 2016933389

Published by Nova Science Publishers, Inc. † New York

CONTENTS

PREFACE

Physiological functions of the body (muscle contraction, visceral activities, glandular functions, etc.) are regulated autonomously by a constituent of the peripheral nervous system commonly known as the autonomic nervous system (ANS). The ANS is controlled by centers found in the spinal cord, brain stem and hypothalamus. The authors of this book discuss the clinical features, functions and disorders of the ANS.

Chapter 1 - Fine tuning of the cardiovascular system is regulated by the autonomic nervous system that comprises sympathetic and parasympathetic components with inhibitory and stimulatory effects, respectively. Crosstalk between sympathetic and parasympathetic nerves that are spatially associated in cardiac plexuses and ganglia is stimulated by neurotransmitters or inflammatory cytokines. Under normal circumstances, afferent information from the heart is transmitted through different hierarchal levels of the nervous system. Heart disease is believed to involve the interplay between neurohumoral, cardiomyocyte and structural elements. Recent studies suggest that an imbalance between the major components of the autonomic nervous system could be critical for disease progression. The authors discuss recent literature from animal models and clinical studies regarding the regulation of myocardial blood flow and ventricular function following surgical disconnection of the heart from the extra-cardiac nervous system. In addition, the authors summarize current knowledge regarding development of post-ischemic tissue injury after cardiac decentralization and examine the potential importance of intact cardiac nerves on organ protection strategies. Future studies using an integrative approach should help to improve understanding of underlying physiopathological mechanisms and eventual development of optimal clinical strategies for management of risk associated with cardiovascular disease.

Chapter 2 - As is well known, the respective function of autonomic nervous system is at least partly responsible for anybody´s individual risk. In that concern it can be supposed by a series of investigations that the vagal part of autonomic function is more sensible reacting to noxious effects than the sympathetic one. Corresponding coherence is given by the more rapid recovery of sympathetic drive when autonomic function was formerly suppressed in general. Conversely, in time course of impairment as well when toxic effects will become stronger, the sympathetic response will become relatively more depressed than the parasympathetic one. This may explain that global parameters of heart rate variability (HRV), for example, sometimes had greater prognostic relevance than information upon spectral analysis. As such, the ratio of special components may lead to inconsistent figures when valuation will be performed too much overall and without differentiation.

With respect to such complex coherences, additional hints are getting to more interest that particularly a reduced vagal function or the herewith furthermore reduced anti-inflammation and NO delivery should be responsible for a lot of complications. Such are elevating the risk for premature death. Therefore, one must be aware that beyond autonomic function in general especially vagal parts of autonomic nervous system should not be stressed unnecessarily. Anticholinergic effects without medical indication should be avoided if possible. On the other side it could be also demonstrated that the prognosis can be improved in several circumstances when vagal influences will become intentionally elevated. However, until now this was only found by electrical vagus nerve stimulation. Nevertheless, in this concern can be thoroughly assumed that the pharmacological potential should be promising as well, but surely more by the precondition that the respective aim corridor is known.

This hypothesis will be underlined if the authors look, for example, at the pleiotropic profile of (1) beta blockers, (2) statins and (3) metformin. All those agents is common (1) that they are reducing cardiovascular risks, (2) that they are reducing the incidence or severity of bacterial infections and (3) that they are also positively influencing cancer diseases regarding to lower incidence and progress. Consequently, (4) mortality was lower found in many studies even without further differentiation when these agents were given before. Furthermore is striking that in all three cases either the vagal activity in heart rate variability (HRV) analysis was found to increase or the sympathetic activity in muscle sympathetic nerve activity (MSNA) was found to decrease.

Thus, one should really surprise that the aspect of functional alteration is not adequately taken into pharmacological consideration, especially if the safety of drugs or the advantage in comparison of drugs is concerned.

Likewise is not adequately realized that metformin, for example, is not only reducing the blood glucose and the mortality in general as well, but has furthermore positive effects (1) in different cancer diseases, (2) in different liver diseases, (3) in intestinal inflammation, (4) in rheumatoid arthritis and additionally (5) in diverse neurological diseases like Parkinson´s disease, multiple sclerosis, some forms of dementia, epilepsy and in ischemic stroke as well. (6) Furthermore, the risk of cognition decline was mostly reduced in diabetes. Regarding to autonomic function changes, today is already known that in most of patient groups mentioned above is typical that they are influenced by a diminished autonomic response, especially in the vagal determined part. And that all metformin effects should be exclusively referred to defined cell-biological or biochemical mechanisms is not even very probable. More unspecific influences should be also considered, surely at least as an environmental co-factor. Such can be improved by drugs but - more often - aggravated by drugs.

The existence of such unspecific but relevant effects will be underlined by the fact that, for example, any alcohol consume is elevating the incidence of infection and cancer, and the last, although invitro no increased cancerogenity was found until now. The coherences were only found and confirmed on the ground of retrospective observations. Furthermore is to consider that autonomic functions, for example, in diabetics and in patients with neurological diseases are typically changed similarly to alcohol dependent subjects. Analogously, elevated incidences of infection and cancer were often seen in such patient groups. Just inverse are the observational findings upon physical activity where specific molecular effects should be nearly excluded. Similar holds true for psychical stress, sleep deprivation, noise and air pollution. In this rather a sympathetic predominance or a lastly diminished oxygen supply should be more probable for etiology and pathogenesis.

For the assumption that more relevant unspecific effects may act on autonomic and immunologic level is also speaking that not only infections but also malignant diseases were more often ascertained (1) by the use of newer antidiabetics when are compared with metformin - as well as (2) when patients are receiving anesthesia or analgesia/sedation as well as (3) after application of erythrocyte concentrates. All could be well explained by a measurable reduction of autonomic/immunologic function.

On the ground of the above-discussed considerations the presented paper engaged on different aspects upon the autonomic modulation of physical functions and here especially on vagal parts. It is summarized (1) what is evidence from the literature, (2) what can be supposed by the existing data and (3) where may be potentials for practical use in the future. Accordingly, not only HRV analysis and MSNA are focused, moreover other non-invasive alternatives like pulse wave velocity, oxygen saturation or blood glucose variation are mentioned. On the other side diverse conflicting interests that are opposing against such investigations are nominated as well.

Chapter 3 - Most of the time, we do not have a good level of awareness of the overall state of our own health. Nor do the authors necessarily want others to know about it if we know that we are in poor health. However, there currently exists neither an objective scale nor satisfactory terminology to describe an individual's general state of health, which makes it difficult to articulate. For this reason, the author studied non-verbal communication of individuals' physiological condition during periods of unconsciousness – i.e., during sleep.

In daily life we accept various services, and the suppliers thereof usually want to know to what extent customers were satisfied with the services provided. However, a range of constraints mean that the authors do not always provide an honest response. Moreover, customers are sometimes unaware of services accepted. In questionnaire responses, for example, the customer's feedback vis-à-vis services received is, for various reasons, often distorted. The same is true of cases pertaining to health and satisfaction, and problems may be caused by mental activity, i.e., consciousness. The notion of entrusting the response to a service to the autonomic nervous system during sleep has therefore been suggested and demonstrated.

It is known that both respiration and pulse during sleep are controlled by the autonomic nervous system. To investigate respiration and pulse, a pressure sensor was used. The pressure signal was conceptualized as the body motion wave (BMW). As well as enabling a broader understanding of the autonomic nervous system, this method also enabled investigation of sleeping posture and body action. The method was initially confirmed using stimuli of aroma and music, since these are known to be conducive to relaxation. The autonomic nervous system responded to the relaxation effect (satisfaction) with a decrease in respiration and pulse rates. The same method was then applied to evaluation of other services, e.g., bedding materials, both on the market and those in development, to gather data on the autonomic nervous system's responses. These materials were thus classified according to satisfaction as expressed by physical activity rather than mental activity.

On the basis of this study, more of control was studied. It was found that the respiratory and cardiovascular systems are controlled in a different manner during periods of increase and decrease. Linked to this, changes in sleeping posture occur not in a random order but, as it were, in a physiological order, that is, a trigger to increase or decrease respiration and/or pulse rate rapidly in a wide range. Subsequently, the question of why and how the rate increases and decreases periodically was investigated by studying the instantaneous pulse rate. The results indicate that the pulse rate does not remain constant, but varies, with roughly three pulse rate ranges per minute, and fluctuates significantly at both higher and lower rate ranges.

Chapter 1

IMPLICATION OF AUTONOMIC NERVOUS SYSTEM DYSFUNCTION ON PATHOGENESIS OF MYOCARDIAL INJURY AND PROTECTION

John G. Kingma[*], *Denis Simard and Jacques R. Rouleau*
Department of Medicine, Faculty of Medicine, Laval Unversity,
Ville de Québec, Canada

ABSTRACT

Fine tuning of the cardiovascular system is regulated by the autonomic nervous system that comprises sympathetic and parasympathetic components with inhibitory and stimulatory effects, respectively. Crosstalk between sympathetic and parasympathetic nerves that are spatially associated in cardiac plexuses and ganglia is stimulated by neurotransmitters or inflammatory cytokines. Under normal circumstances, afferent information from the heart is transmitted through different hierarchal levels of the nervous system. Heart disease is believed to involve the interplay between neurohumoral, cardiomyocyte and structural elements. Recent studies suggest that an imbalance between the major components of the autonomic nervous system could be critical for disease progression. We discuss recent literature from animal models and clinical studies regarding the regulation of myocardial blood flow and ventricular function following surgical disconnection of the heart from the extra-cardiac nervous system. In addition, we summarize

---

[*] Corresponding author: Email: john.kingma@fmed.ulaval.ca.

current knowledge regarding development of post-ischemic tissue injury after cardiac decentralization and examine the potential importance of intact cardiac nerves on organ protection strategies. Future studies using an integrative approach should help to improve understanding of underlying physiopathological mechanisms and eventual development of optimal clinical strategies for management of risk associated with cardiovascular disease.

Keywords: autonomic nervous system, sympathetic, parasympathetic nerves, intrinsic cardiac neurons, vasoregulation, ischemia, reperfusion, organ conditioning, inter-organ crosstalk

INTRODUCTION

Physiological functions of the body (muscle contraction, visceral activities, glandular functions, etc.) are regulated autonomously by a constituent of the peripheral nervous system commonly known as the autonomic nervous system. The autonomic nervous system is controlled by centers found in the spinal cord, brain stem and hypothalamus. Two interacting systems - sympathetic and parasympathetic – either stimulate energy expenditure under conditions of stress (i.e., fight or flight) or return the body to a restful state. Both sympathetic and parasympathetic pathways consist of preganglionic and postganglionic neurons that are activated by different endogenous chemical neurotransmitters. Increasing attention is focused on the complex anatomy and function of the cardiac neuroaxis. How different populations of neurons within peripheral autonomic and intrathoracic ganglia communicate with each other, and between different organ systems, remains an open question. This chapter reviews recent scientific literature and experimental initiatives including those from our laboratory that have examined the role of intrinsic cardiac neurons on regulation of myocardial blood flow, pre- and post-ischemic cardiac function, development of tissue injury without and with organ conditioning pretreatment and inter-organ crosstalk.

ANATOMY OF THE INTRATHORACIC NERVOUS SYSTEM

Several important phases have been described for development of autonomic heart nerves; 1) migration of neural crest cells to the dorsal aorta, 2) differentiation of neural crest cells to neurons, 3) migration of neurons to form either paravertebral sympathetic chains or parasympathetic cardiac ganglia, 4) extension of axonal projections into cardiac tissue and terminal differentiation [66]. The sympathetic component of the autonomic nervous system stimulates cardiac conduction and myocardial cells while the parasympathetic exerts an inhibitory influence [86, 112]. Sympathetic cardiac nerves originate from stellate, the superior, middle cervical and thoracic ganglia [66]. Postganglionic sympathetic neurons project efferent axons across various areas of the heart [46]; however, their development differs with respect to degree and density. Parasympathetic nerves evolve from the cardiac component of the cranial neural crest; primary access of preganglionic neurons to the heart occurs via both vagus nerves [43, 60]. Cardiac ganglia are located discretely within the atrial epicardium associated with epicardial fat, within ganglionated plexi along the major cardiac vessels and within the ventricular wall [4, 93, 102]. The number and location of cardiac ganglia varies between species depending on body size and heart activity [67]. Neurons within the autonomic nervous system are characterized by chemical phenotyping; cholinergic and adrenergic populations of ganglionic cardiac neurons are readily found within cardiac ganglia [47, 103, 114]. Sensory neurons, interneurons and sensory fibers originating from the *nucleus ambiguous* have also been found here [2, 6, 75] and are likely to play a role in physiopathological processes and pathogenesis of cardiac disease. Regulation of cardiac function in health and disease are likely to be affected by status of the cardiac nervous system and the interactions between central command (i.e., brainstem) and the intrinsic cardiac neurons (Figure 1) on the heart (sometimes referred to as the 'little brain on the heart' [7]) [21, 57]. Indeed, the intrinsic cardiac nervous system comprises all neuronal elements essential for intracardiac reflex control and is independent of higher centers [78, 91]. As such, despite altered connectivity neurons within this system generate spontaneous activity to regulate regional cardiac function reflexively. This is most evident in the setting of cardiac transplantation [13].

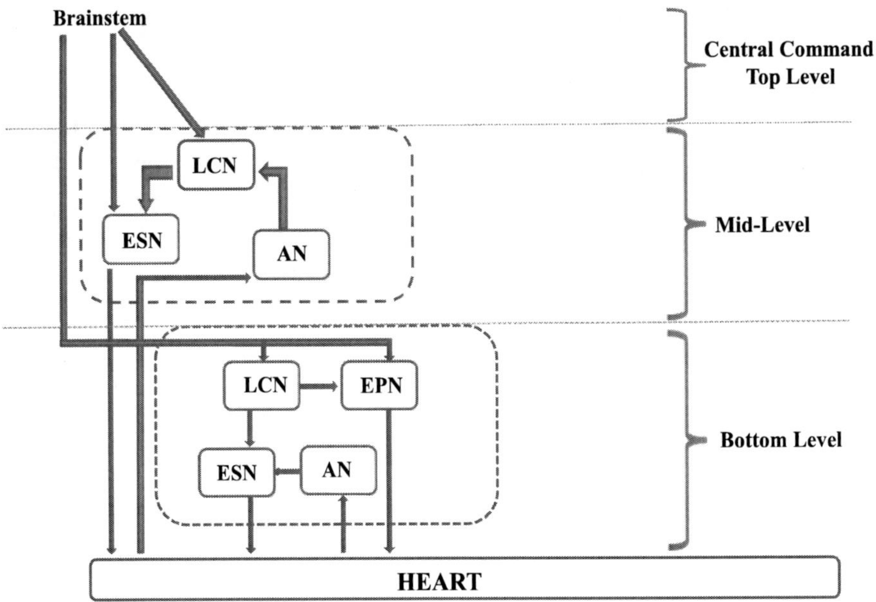

Figure 1. Schematic organisation of cardiac innervation between the central nervous system and the heart. LCN: local circuit neurons, ESN: efferent sympathetic neurons, AN: afferent neurons, EPN: efferent parasympathetic neurons.

Reliable animal models of surgical decentralization (this term is used rather than denervation because the heart is simply disconnected from central command (Figure 2) and ganglionated plexi on the heart and surrounding tissue are not removed) to study reflex control of heart function have been developed. In this model the heart is completely decentralized from central command as evidenced by the lack of sympathetic/parasympathetic responses to extracardiac stimulation [69] and as such is analogous to the transplanted denervated heart [22, 36]. Chemical sympathectomy by phenol painting of connective and neural tissues around the ascending aorta, left pulmonary vein and main pulmonary artery has also been used [93, 95]. Likewise, pharmacologic agents (reserpine, 6-hydroxydopamine, hexamethonium, etc.) can be used to block interneuron communications; however, they have the disadvantage of peripheral secondary effects [17, 92, 104].

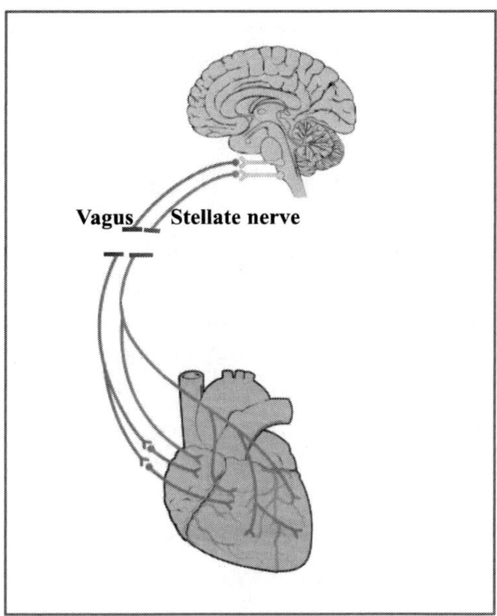

Figure 2. Schematic of surgical intervention for decentralization of the heart from central command.

INTRINSIC CARDIAC NEURONS AND VASOREGULATION

Though coronary blood flow is primarily regulated by local metabolic changes, the autonomic nervous system also plays a major role. Stimulation of sympathetic nerves initiates a biphasic response (vasoconstriction followed by vasodilatation) that trends to coronary dilatation due to increases in myocardial oxygen consumption and perfusion pressure. Local administration of neuropeptides indirectly affects distribution of blood flow across the ventricular wall by modulating cardiac dynamics [8, 18, 61]; however, local increases in catecholamine levels also stimulate sympathetic fibers.

Published findings on the effects of cardiac decentralization on blood flow regulation vary considerably [26, 39, 111]. Vergroesen and co-workers documented (i.e., cardiac denervation model) a role for cardiac nerves with regard to the speed of response of the coronary vascular bed to changes in heart rate and perfusion pressure [111]. In a canine cardiac decentralization model, we showed that cardiac neurons could function independently of central neuronal inputs with respect to coronary autoregulation; we also reported that the leftward shift of the coronary artery pressure-flow relation that occurs after blockade of angiotensin II receptors was not affected by ablation of extracardiac nerves [97]. However, subtle complications within the microvasculature at different levels across the ventricular wall could also influence myocardial autoregulation and cell viability. For instance, Rimoldi and co-workers revealed that regional sympathetic denervation did not affect either baseline or hyperemic myocardial blood flow within denervated areas (vs. innervated areas) [95]. Since ventricular blood flow at baseline is nearly uniform [12] they suggested that 1) homeostasis of blood flow could be maintained by a combination of neural modulation and autoregulation principally at the microvascular level, and 2) a shift in coronary resistance through autoregulatory adjustments within microvessels less than 100 μm in diameter. However, these factors could be less relevant when vessels are maximally vasodilated. During hyperemia, the innervation/ventricular perfusion relation in neuropathy patients has been shown to be lower in innervated regions but is unaffected within denervated myocardium [105]. These findings contrast with results from human subjects that showed a significantly higher hyperemic blood flow after suppression of adenosine-mediated sympathetic activation [55].

In heart transplant recipients higher blood flow during sympathetic stimulation appears to be correlated with norepinephrine levels in cardiac sympathetic nerve terminals [26]; resting coronary flow in these patients appears not to be affected by humoral or neural adrenergic influences. Other studies report that coronary flow reserve in transplant recipients is not altered by pharmacologic blockade of α- or β-adrenergic receptors [45].

Neuromodulation treatments such as spinal cord stimulation (SCS) are currently being used to treat various clinical syndromes such as congestive heart failure, cancer related pain and chronic pain, etc. SCS activates spinal cord neurons by bioelectrical modulation that produces a conformational change within the intrinsic cardiac nervous system; during ischemia, this remodeling can override excitatory inputs from the affected myocardium and provoke regional cardiac electrical and mechanical effects. Application of SCS activates sensory afferent fibers via the release of endogenous neuropeptides which, in turn, affect activity of intrinsic cardiac neurons [32]. In patients with progressive vascular disease, SCS has been shown to improve myocardial perfusion reserve and distribution of myocardial blood flow. In addition, SCS augmented the blood flow response (due to sympathetic stimulation of endothelium-mediated vasodilatation) to cold-pressor tests which suggests an amelioration of vasomotor function [99]; however, it remains unclear that these improvements persist for prolonged periods.

INTRINSIC CARDIAC NEURONS AND ISCHEMIA-RELATED INJURY

Understanding the physiopathological mechanisms that are solicited within the neuronal hierarchy which regulates post-ischemic cardiac function remains a significant challenge. Involvement of autonomic neurons in cardiac regulation depends on their location within the myocardium and the response characteristics of their sensory inputs. Sympathetic and parasympathetic nerves in the left ventricle are localized near cardiac myocytes to permit rapid crosstalk [20] – loss of this crosstalk could potentially influence myocyte responses to ischemia. Modulation of intrinsic cardiac neurons by myocardial ischemia occurs subsequent to limited oxygen availability and energy substrates and is potentially due to local accumulation of metabolic by-products such as reactive oxygen species and purinergic compounds [48, 50, 106]. Though considerable effort has been made to find ways to protect cardiocytes from ischemic injury only a handful of studies have addressed the question of whether reperfusion of the infarct-related coronary vessel directly influences neuron activity within the infarct risk area. Nerves that course over, or through, infarcted myocardium could be functionally impaired due to compromised blood flow [10]. Some evidence suggests that the blood supply of these nerves is little affected by local ischemic conditions thereby permitting these nerves to conduct action potentials [52]. On the other hand, restoration of blood flow to necrotic regions of the ventricular wall does not insure against further complications. Recent animal and human studies that have addressed the subject of ischemic injury and autonomic nervous system are highlighted in Table 1.

Whether intrinsic cardiac neurons are more, or less sensitive to ischemic, or reperfusion damage compared to cardiocytes remains an open question; the injury threshold of cardiac neurons also remains a subject of debate and needs to be established. Furthermore, Arora and Armour examined cardiac neuron activity during myocardial ischemia and reperfusion in a porcine model [9]; they showed that responsiveness of ventricular neurons to distal ischemia was due to the sum of inputs from multiple ventricular sensory neurites capable of transducing mechanical and chemical milieu of the ventricle. For instance, adenosine (catabolite produced during ischemia) stimulates neurons in the central nervous system and autonomic ganglia in the heart [3] and sympathetic efferent postganglionic axons that innervate coronary vessels [1]. Oxygen free radicals also stimulate ventricular sensory neurites [106]. As such, ischemia affects the hierarchy of signal transduction between intrinsic cardiac and ventricular neurons. Arora and Armour documented that adenosine-induced responses of intrinsic cardiac neurons are obtunded during ischemia but can be restored during reperfusion (after washout from ischemic zone) [9].

During cardiac ischemia sympathetic efferents are activated and catecholamines are discharged within the ischemic myocardium (independently of the central sympathetic nervous system) [77, 108]. Catecholamines modulate myocardial oxygen demand, intracellular calcium overload, arrhythmias and cellular necrosis; however, studies in rabbits subject to acute blockade of efferent cardiac sympathetic nerves did not show significant infarct limiting effects [41, 107]. Finally, neuronal impairment might also extend to areas outside the under-perfused zone or area of necrosis [10, 25].

Table 1. Intrinsic cardiac nerves and myocardial ischemia

Study	Study goals	Study Design	Main Results
Basic research			
Calvillo et al. [19]	• to determine if vagal stimulation (VS) modulates inflammation after acute myocardial ischemia	• infarct size, inflammation and apoptosis evaluated after 30-min ischemia and 24h reperfusion in rats • 3 groups treated with VS and compared to controls	• VS decreases infarct size and inflammatory markers • anti-inflammatory and anti-apoptotic properties of the nicotinic pathway
Kingma et al. [62]	• intact cardiac nervous system involved in ischemic injury	• infarct size evaluated after 60-min ischemia and 180-min reperfusion in cardiac decentralized dogs	• ischemic injury not exacerbated in decentralized heart
Nguyen et al. [82]	• to examine if myocardial ischemia induces bilateral stellate ganglia nerve sprouting	• rabbits subject to acute myocardial ischemia • magnitude of nerve sprouting evaluated using immunohistochemistry	• myocardial infarction increases serum nerve growth factor levels and induces nerve sprouting and hyperinnervation (adrenergic and cholinergic axons) in the stellate ganglia

Study	Study goals	Study Design	Main Results
Clinical research			
Werner et al. [115]	• to investigate regional sympathetic nerve damage and restoration in rats subject to transient myocardial ischemia	• rats subject to transient ischemia and reperfusion • dual-tracer autoradiography performed at 7 days and 2 months post-ischemia	• higher susceptibility of sympathetic neurons compared to myocytes to ischemia • partial re-innervation in subepicardium within ischemic zone
Lujan et al. [73]	• to investigate novel strategies for prevention of sudden cardiac death	• cholera toxin B subunit conjugated to saporin injected into stellate ganglia before being subjected to ischemia in rats	• ablation of cardiac sympathetic neurons reduces susceptibility to ventricular arrhythmias
Saraste et al. [99]	• to examine effects of spinal cord stimulation (SCS) therapy on ischemic tolerance and myocardial perfusion reserve	• SCS in patients (n = 18) with refractory angina pectoris • blood flow evaluated by PET during adenosine stress	• short term SCS increases ischemic tolerance, perfusion reserve and endothelium-mediated vasomotor function in advanced coronary artery disease
Kawasaki et al. [56]	• to determine if Bezold-Jarisch reflex or enhancement of vagal nerves results after exercise ischemia	• exercise myocardial scintigraphy and coronary angiography performed in patients (n = 145) • heart rate variability examined	• vagal modulation increased in association with exercise induced inferoposterior ischemia

Neuropeptide release by sensory neurites also modulates activity of intrinsic cardiac neurons [8, 24]. Axon damage produced by ischemia affects neuropeptide production in sympathetic neurons which innervate the heart [40]. Even after ischemia, cardiac sympathetic neurons could be functionally competent; this notion is supported by the finding of higher galanin (promotes regeneration of sympathetic axons) levels in cardiac sympathetic neurons post-ischemia. In addition, galanin is known to modify synaptic transmission and thereby contribute to cardiac arrhythmias and sudden cardiac death. Other autacoids (adenosine, bradykinin) along with nitric oxide and oxygen free radicals that trigger intracellular signal transduction in various cell types are released during ischemia and can initiate responses in somata and axons of the mammalian intrinsic cardiac nervous system [7].

Ardell and co-workers recently examined functional remodeling of neuronal elements post-infarction in pigs and reported that: 1) intracardiac ganglia undergo morphological and phenotypic remodeling depending on the site of injury; 2) afferent neural signals to intracardiac neurons in ischemic tissue are attenuated but those from border and remote regions are preserved thereby creating a « *neural sensory border zone* » between injured and non-injured myocardium; 3) autonomic efferent inputs to the intrinsic cardiac nervous system are maintained; 4) transduction capacity is augmented in convergent intrinsic cardiac local circuit neurons (that receive afferent and efferent inputs) and 5) functional network connectivity of intrinsic cardiac neurons is significantly reduced [91]. More importantly, they reported that neural remodeling was independent of direct ischemic injury to a specific subset of neurons. Plasticity of neurons within the cardiac neuraxis is considered crucial during evolution of cardiac disease or post-infarction [34, 42]. Healed myocardium post-infarction provides a particular challenge to electrical propagation and thereby integrative regulation of cardiac function [98, 110]. In this setting a continual state of abnormal cardiac afferent signaling exists that leads to continuous discord between central and peripheral aspects of the neural hierarchy; this leads to a scenario of excessive sympathoexcitation resulting in fatal arrhythmias [34]. Autonomic regulation therapies including cardiac afferent denervation and sympathectomy (for ventricular tachycardia) have been attributed to the reduction of conflict between different levels within the hierarchy of the cardiac nervous system [15, 58]. As such, it is noteworthy that the intrinsic nervous system of the heart is able to preserve neural coordination and electrical stability even in the absence of inputs from higher central command; a clear example of this principle is transplanted heart [109].

Information processing within the central nervous system has also been examined using targeted SCS; in the heart, SCS appears to reduce excitability of intrinsic cardiac neurons and stabilize cardiac function and may protect against deleterious consequences of ischemia. Several studies have documented that activity of intrinsic cardiac neurons is increased during ischemia and reperfusion that induces ventricular arrhythmias or even fibrillation [49, 51].

INTRINSIC CARDIAC NEURONS AND ORGAN CONDITIONING

Organ conditioning (direct, remote anesthetic, pharmacologic, non-pharmacologic) as a preventive strategy for tissue protection against ischemic injury has been the focus of numerous animal and human investigations since 1986 (cf. Table 2). In the heart, endogenous protection against ischemia-reperfusion injury by ischemic preconditioning (IPc) was first described in canine studies from the Reimer laboratory [79]. Two distinct windows of protection by IPc have been defined [89, 90, 116] but the underlying mechanisms have not been clearly identified. In their seminal study, Przyklenk and co-workers [88] demonstrated that repetitive non-lethal ischemia of the left circumflex artery vascular bed mitigated cellular injury in the adjacent vascular bed (i.e., left anterior descending artery) that was subjected to prolonged ischemia. This particular study initiated the concept of «preconditioning at a distance» or «remote conditioning» which has been the subject of numerous experimental and clinical studies. Remote conditioning (Rc) may be the most clinically relevant non-pharmacologic strategy for organ protection against ischemic injury.

Neural and humoral pathways stimulate endogenous cellular pathways in response to acute ischemic injury. Within the current paradigm, preconditioning stimulates endogenous ligands (adenosine, opioids, etc.) and catecholamines that trigger intracellular transduction pathways to mediate cytoprotective end-effectors (from cell surface to the mitochondria) to initiate protection [44, 116]. An intriguing unanswered aspect of organ conditioning stratagems revolves around the question of how cytoprotective signals are transmitted; several pathways worthy of consideration include 1) communication via blood or perfusate borne humoral factors, 2) communication by neuronal stimulation, and 3) communication by systemic alteration of circulating immune cells [27, 100, 113]. Potential candidate molecules released from ischemic tissues that interact with receptors to trigger a cytoprotective response remain to be identified. A number of studies in isolated non-preconditioned hearts perfused with buffer collected from preconditioned hearts have reported significant tissue protection [16, 27]. Protective factors have been identified as thermolabile hydrophobic compounds with molecular weights <30 kDa [68, 101]; at least one of these compounds has been suggested to initiate cytoprotection via stimulation of intracellular signalling pathways (i.e., PI3K/Akt-dependent, RISK, SAFE, etc.)

[16, 71, 94]. Whether these compounds stimulate intrinsic cardiac nerves has not been resolved.

Table 2. Intrinsic cardiac neurons and remote conditioning

Study	Study goals	Study Design	Main Results
Basic research			
Basalay et al. [11]	• to study involvement of neural and humoral mechanisms for remote conditioning (Rc)	• rats subject to ischemia/reperfusion (CO/RP) • capsaicin SC at 25-min before CO, 25-min after CO, 10-min after RP • bilateral sectioning of femoral and sciatic nerves before CO • vagotomy before CO	• Rc induced cardioprotection requires afferent innervation of the remote organ • intact parasympathetic activity required for Rc protection • signalling pathways are involved in delayed Rc
Redington et al. [94]	• to study the role of femoral nerve stimulation on induction of Rc protection	• rabbits pretreated by Rc • dialysate collected and added to perfusate • Langendorff preparation – hearts subject to CO/RP	• direct electrical/peripheral neural stimulation promotes release of endogenous protective compounds into the bloodstream that limit ischemic injury
Donato et al. [28]	• to study participation of vagus nerve and muscarinic receptors in Rc	• rabbits pretreated by Rc • vagal stimulation • sciatic and femoral nerve section • spinal cord section • rabbits subject to CO/RP	• Rc activates neural afferent pathway to stimulate protection • spinal cord section abolished Rc protection • acetylcholine activates Rc via muscarinic receptors
Kingma et al. [63]	• to study whether intact cardiac nerves are required to mediate Rc	• dogs subject to CO/RP • Rc pretreatment in dogs with intact cardiac nerves and after cardiac decentralization	• Rc mediated protection not abrogated by chemical or surgical decentralization
Enko et al. [29]	• to determine if Rc induces vasodilatation in adjacent vascular beds	• changes in arterial diameter evaluated during Rc in healthy patients (n = 20) • power spectral analysis	• vessel dilatation during Rc • parasympathetic activity higher time-dependently during

Study	Study goals	Study Design	Main Results
Basic research			
	• to evaluate autonomic nerve activity during Rc	of heart rate examined	Rc
Loukogeo-rgakis et al. [72]	• characterize time course and neural mechanism of Rc	• endothelial injury measured by flow-mediated dilatation in healthy patients (n = 16) • trimetaphan administered to evaluate neuronal involvement	• two phases of protection against endothelial injury in humans subject to Rc

The role of cardiac nerves in the first window of IPc has not yet been determined; surgical sympathectomy may not affect first window IPc-mediated protection [5, 65]. Findings from our laboratory in dogs pretreated with IPc document that protection against ischemic injury was conserved even after target tissues were disconnected from central command [63]. However, second window IPc is abrogated following cardiac decentralization [65]; these findings could be interpreted to indicate that cellular protection mechanisms are not triggered by neural stimulation. We have also reported significant cardioprotection by Rc in surgically and pharmacologically (i.e., hexamethonium) cardiac decentralized dogs subject to ischemia-reperfusion injury [62, 63]. However, further studies are necessary as blockade of sympathetic and parasympathetic ganglia with systemic hexamethonium appears to abolish Rc mediated organ protection [38, 74]. Additionally, actions of volatile anesthetic agents which stimulate preconditioning pathways [23, 76] on the autonomic nervous system remain to be established.

PERSPECTIVES

Bi-directional interactions between sympathetic and parasympathetic efferent pathways are reported to occur at different levels of the neuraxis and within target organs [85]. There is strong evidence that autonomic nervous system dysfunction contributes to co-morbidities that evolve in different organ systems. Recognition, even at the subclinical level, of early autonomic nervous system dysfunction has been highlighted in several clinical investigations (cf. Table 3) [37, 87]. Diabetes, renal or cardiovascular disease impact significantly on autonomic imbalance and impaired baroreflex function and have been linked to morbidity and mortality in patients. Early subclinical autonomic neuropathy is strongly associated with insulin resistance [70]; in chronic heart failure end-organ damage and neurohumoral activation are believed to contribute to impaired autonomic control. Ewing initially described autonomic dysfunction as reduced nerve conduction velocity and longer terminal latency in patients with abnormal heart rate [30, 31]. During chronic kidney disease, accumulation of uremic toxins have been reported to influence neural conduction parameters [64]; these changes are rapidly reversed with hemodialysis or after kidney transplantation [59, 83, 84]. Non-neural anomalies associated with micro-albuminuria (vascular injury, increased thickness of the tunica media at baroreceptor sites, impaired cardiac vagal function, reduced vessel reactivity, etc.) should also be considered. Additionally, the relation between microvascular disease and autonomic nervous system dysfunction has been emphasized for patients with diabetes and chronic kidney disease but there is no real consensus since microalbuminuria and cardiovascular autonomic dysfunction are independently associated with cardiac-related mortality [14].

The role of the central nervous and autonomic nervous systems on inflammation under physiopathological conditions also remains an open and highly interesting research area; the reader is referred to a Special Issue of Autonomic Neuroscience: Basic and Clinical published in 2014 that addresses current questions concerning the autonomic nervous system and inflammation. Sympatho-neural and sympatho-adrenal systems regulate protective mechanisms at both the cellular and organ levels. Noxious stimuli activate primary afferent nociceptive neurons and the central nociceptive system which trigger various actions via the autonomic nervous and neuroendocrine systems to coordinate a protective response at the cellular level [53, 54]. Overproduction of inflammatory cytokines during organ injury (all cause) invariably activates inflammatory pathways and cellular protective mechanisms. Inflammation encompasses two distinct phases (i.e., development and resolution phases) that are finely coordinated [81]; the central nervous and immune systems communicate via primary afferent nociceptive neurons that are found in most body tissues and cytokines that are released from different immune cells or lymphoid organs. Neural communication between the brain and immune system is believed to occur via distinct sympathetic pathways not related to other peripheral sympathetic pathways including vasoconstrictor, visceral secretomotor or visceral motility-regulatory systems [54].

Table 3. Co-morbidities and intrinsic cardiac nerves

Study	Study goals	Study Design	Main Results
Clinical research			
Gaudreault et al. [35]	• to study association between exercise-induced hypertension and heart rate variability in men with metabolic syndrome (MetS).	• blood pressure measured before, during and after treadmill test (n = 98) • insulin resistance and oral glucose tests performed	• normotensive men with MetS have greater insulin resistance and lower heart rate variability parasympathetic/sympathetic indices.
Rosengard-Barlund et al. [96]	• to evaluate baroreflex sensitivity in normal and type 1 diabetic patients with autonomic dysfunction	• autonomic function tests (n = 152; 116 diabetes type 1 and 36 healthy controls) • spectral analysis of heart rate and blood pressure variability • baroreflex sensitivity estimated at baseline, slow deep-breathing and supine and standing positions	• increased sympathetic activity in patients with type 1 diabetes • early autonomic derangements are functional and potentially correctable
Franchitto et al. [33]	• to evaluate if cardiorenal anemia syndrome (CRAS) in chronic heart failure (CHF) patients contributes to sympathetic over activity	• muscle sympathetic nerve activity compared in patients with CRAS + CHF (n = 15) and matched controls (n = 15) • sympathetic baroreflex function also evaluated	• CRAS in CHF patients increases sympathetic activity due to tonic activation of peripheral and baroreflex impairment
Study	**Study goals**	**Study Design**	**Main Results**
Nasr et al. [80]	• to assess the association between cardiovascular autonomic neuropathy (CAN) and impaired cerebral autoregulation in patients with type 1 diabetes	• dynamic cerebral autoregulation (DCA) evaluated using transcranial Doppler (n = 60) • CAN defined on basis of heart rate variability during deep breathing, Valsalva manoeuver or initiation of active standing	• CAN associated with DCA in type 1 diabetes • level of DCA impairment increased in relation to severity of CAN

The autonomic nervous system appears to play an essential role in inter-organ crosstalk pathways. Re-organisation of inter-organ communication pathways after organ injury may be the determining factor for survival. Future studies using an integrative approach (i.e., immunology, inflammation, autonomic nervous system, nociception and pain, cellular protection and regulation of organ function) should help to improve understanding of underlying physiopathological mechanisms and eventual development of optimal therapeutic interventions.

REFERENCES

[1]   Abe, T., Morgan, D. A. and Gutterman, D. D. (1997). Role of adenosine receptor subtypes in neural stunning of sympathetic coronary innervation. *Am J Physiol (Heart Circ Physiol)*, *272*, H25-H34.

[2]   Ai, J., Epstein, PN., Gozal, D., Yang, B., Wurster, R. and Cheng, Z. J. (2007). Morphology and topography of nucleus ambiguus projections to cardiac ganglia in rats and mice. *Neuroscience*, *149*, 845-860.

[3]   Allen, T. G. J. and Burnstock, G. (1990). The actions of adenosine 5'-triphosphate on guinea-pig intracardiac neurones in culture. *Br J Pharmacol, 100*, 269-276.

[4]   Ardell, J. L. and Randall, W. C. (1986). Selective vagal innervation of sinoatrial and atrioventricular nodes in canine heart. *Am J Physiol (Heart Circ Physiol)*, *251*, H764-H773.

[5]   Ardell, J. L., Yang, X. M., Barron, B. A., Downey, J. M. and Cohen, M. V. (1996). Endogenous myocardial norepinephrine is not essential for ischemic preconditioning in rabbit heart. *Am J Physiol (Heart Circ Physiol)*, *270*, H1078-H1084.

[6]   Armour, J. A. (1999). Myocardial ischaemia and the cardiac nervous system. *Cardiovasc Res, 41*, 41-54.

[7]   Armour, J. A. (2008). Potential clinical relevance of the 'little brain' on the mammalian heart. *Exp Physiol*, *93*, 165-176.

[8]   Armour, J. A., Huang, M. H. and Smith, F. M. (1993). Peptidergic modulation of *in situ* canine intrinsic cardiac neurons. *Peptides*, *14*, 191-202.

[9]   Arora, R. C. and Armour, J. A. (2003). Adenosine A1 receptor activation reduces myocardial reperfusion effects on intrinsic cardiac nervous system. *Am J Physiol Regul Integr Comp Physiol*, *284*, R1314-R1321.

[10] Barber, M. J., Mueller, T. M., Henry, D. P., Felten, S. Y. and Zipes, D. P. (1983). Transmural myocardial infarction in the dog produces sympathectomy in noninfarcted myocardium. *Circ*, *67*, 787-796.

[11] Basalay, M., Barsukevich, V., Mastitskaya, S., Mrochek, A., Pernow, J., Sjoquist, P. O., Ackland, G. L., Gourine, A. V. and Gourine, A. (2012). Remote ischaemic pre- and delayed postconditioning - similar degree of cardioprotection but distinct mechanisms. *Exp Physiol*, *97*, 908-917.

[12] Bassingthwaighte, J. B. (1977). Physiology and theory of tracer washout techniques for the estimation of myocardial blood flow: flow estimation from tracer washout. *Prog Cardiovasc Dis*, *20*, 165-189.

[13] Beckers, F., Ramaekers, D., Speijer, G., Ector, H., Vanhaecke, J., Verheyden, B., Van, C. J., Droogne, W., Van de Werf, F. and Aubert, A. E. (2004). Different evolutions in heart rate variability after heart transplantation: 10-year follow-up. *Transplantation*, *78*, 1523-1531.

[14] Beijers, H. J., Ferreira, I., Bravenboer, B., Dekker, J. M., Nijpels, G., Heine, R. J. and Stehouwer, C. D. (2009). Microalbuminuria and cardiovascular autonomic dysfunction are independently associated with cardiovascular mortality: evidence for distinct pathways: the Hoorn Study. *Diabetes Care*, *32*, 1698-1703.

[15] Bourke, T., Vaseghi, M., Michowitz, Y., Sankhla, V., Shah, M., Swapna, N., Boyle, N. G., Mahajan, A., Narasimhan, C., Lokhandwala, Y. and Shivkumar, K. (2010). Neuraxial modulation for refractory ventricular arrhythmias: value of thoracic epidural anesthesia and surgical left cardiac sympathetic denervation. *Circulation*, *121*, 2255-2262.

[16] Breivik, L., Helgeland, E., Aarnes, E. K., Mrdalj, J. and Jonassen, A. K. (2011). Remote postconditioning by humoral factors in effluent from ischemic preconditioned rat hearts is mediated via PI3K/Akt-dependent cell-survival signaling at reperfusion. *Basic Res Cardiol*, *106*, 135-145.

[17] Brunsting, J. R., Schuil, H. A. and Zijlstra, W. G. (1983). Intrinsic heart rate in the dog determined by pharmacologic denervation. *Am J Physiol*, *245*, H592-H597.

[18] Butler, C. K., Smith, F. M., Cardinal, R., Murphy, D. A. and Hopkins, D. A. (1990). Cardiac responses to electrical stimulation of discrete loci in atrial and ventricular ganglionated plexi. *Am J Physiol (Heart Circ Physiol)*, *259*, H1365-H1373.

[19] Calvillo, L., Vanoli, E., Andreoli, E., Besana, A., Omodeo, E., Gnecchi, M., Zerbi, P., Vago, G., Busca, G. and Schwartz, P. J. (2011). Vagal stimulation, through its nicotinic action, limits infarct size and the

inflammatory response to myocardial ischemia and reperfusion. *J Cardiovasc Pharmacol*, *58*, 500-507.

[20] Canty, J. M. Jr. and Fallavollita, J. A. (2003). Sympathetic nerves and myocyte necrosis: more than meets the eye. *Circ Res*, *93*, 796-798.

[21] Cardinal, R., Page, P., Vermeulen, M., Ardell, J. L. and Armour, J. A. (2009). Spatially divergent cardiac responses to nicotinic stimulation of ganglionated plexus neurons in the canine heart. *Auton Neurosci*, *145*, 55-62.

[22] Chowdhary, S., Harrington, D., Bonser, R. S., Coote, J. H. and Townend, J. N. (2002). Chronotropic effects of nitric oxide in the denervated human heart. *J Physiol*, *541*, 645-651.

[23] Cope, D. K., Impastato, W. K., Cohen, M. V. and Downey, J. M. (1997). Volatile anesthetics protect the ischemic rabbit myocardium from infarction. *Anesthesiology*, *86*, 699-709.

[24] Croom, J. E., Foreman, R. D., Chandler, M. J. and Barron, K. W. (1997). Cutaneous vasodilation during dorsal column stimulation is mediated by dorsal roots and CGRP. *Am J Physiol*, *272*, H950-H957.

[25] Dae, M. W., Herre, J. M., O'Connell, J. W., Botvinick, E. H., Newman, D. and Munoz, L. (1991). Scintigraphic assessment of sympathetic innervation after transmural versus nontransmural myocardial infarction. *J Am Coll Cardiol*, *17*, 1416-1423.

[26] Di Carli, M. f., Tobes, M. C., Mangner, T., Levine, A. B., Muzik, O., Chakroborty, P. and Levine, T. B. (1997). Effects of cardiac sympathetic innervation on coronary blood flow. *New Engl J Med*, *336*, 1208-1215.

[27] Dickson, E. W., Lorbar, M., Porcaro, W. A., Fenton, R. A., Reinhardt, C. P., Gysembergh, A. and Przyklenk, K. (1999). Rabbit heart can be "preconditioned" via transfer of coronary effluent. *Am J Physiol (Heart Circ Physiol)*, *277*, H2451-H2457.

[28] Donato, M., Buchholz, B., Rodriguez, M., Perez, V., Inserte, J., Garcia-Dorado, D. and Gelpi, R. J. (2013). Role of the parasympathetic nervous system in cardioprotection by remote hindlimb ischaemic preconditioning. *Exp Physiol*, *98*, 425-434.

[29] Enko, K., Nakamura, K., Yunoki, K., Miyoshi, T., Akagi, S., Yoshida, M., Toh, N., Sangawa, M., Nishii, N., Nagase, S., Kohno, K., Morita, H., Kusano, K. F. and Ito, H. (2011). Intermittent arm ischemia induces vasodilatation of the contralateral upper limb. *J Physiol Sci*, *61*, 507-513.

[30] Ewing, D. J., Campbell, I. W., Burt, A. A. and Clarke, B. F. (1973). Vascular reflexes in diabetic autonomic neuropathy. *Lancet*, *2*, 1354-1356.

[31] Ewing, D. J., Campbell, I. W. and Clarke, B. F. (1976). Mortality in diabetic autonomic neuropathy. *Lancet, 1*, 601-603.

[32] Foreman, R. D., Linderoth, B., Ardell, J. L., Barron, K. W., Chandler, M. J., Hull, S. S., Jr. TerHorst, G. J., DeJongste, M. J. L. and Armour, J. A. (2000). Modulation of intrinsic cardiac neurons by spinal cord stimulation: implications for its therapeutic use in angina pectoris. *Cardiovasc Res, 47*, 367-375.

[33] Franchitto, N., Despas, F., Labrunee, M., Vaccaro, A., Lambert, E., Lambert, G., Galinier, M., Senard, J. M. and Pathak, A. (2013). Cardiorenal anemia syndrome in chronic heart failure contributes to increased sympathetic nerve activity. *Int J Cardiol, 168*, 2352-2357.

[34] Fukuda, K., Kanazawa, H., Aizawa, Y., Ardell, J. L. and Shivkumar, K. (2015). Cardiac innervation and sudden cardiac death. *Circ Res, 116*, 2005-2019.

[35] Gaudreault, V., Despres, J. P., Rheaume, C., Bergeron, J., Almeras, N., Tremblay, A. and Poirier, P. (2013). Exercise-induced exaggerated blood pressure response in men with the metabolic syndrome: the role of the autonomous nervous system. *Blood Press Monit, 18*, 252-258.

[36] Gerber, B. L., Bernard, X., Melin, J. A., Delestinne, T., Vanbutsele, R., Goenen, M. and Vanoverschelde, J. L. (2001). Exaggerated chronotropic and energetic response to dobutamine after orthotopic cardiac transplantation. *J Heart Lung Transplant, 20*, 824-832.

[37] Gerritsen, J., Dekker, J. M., TenVoorde, B. J., Kostense, P. J., Heine, R. J., Bouter, L. M., Heethaar, R. M. and Stehouwer, C. D. (2001). Impaired autonomic function is associated with increased mortality, especially in subjects with diabetes, hypertension, or a history of cardiovascular disease: the Hoorn Study. *Diabetes Care, 24*, 1793-1798.

[38] Gho, B. C., Schoemaker, R. G., van den Doel, M. A., Duncker, D. J. and Verdouw, P. D. (1996). Myocardial protection by brief ischemia in noncardiac tissue. *Circulation, 94*, 2193-2200.

[39] Gregg, D. E., Khouri, E. M., Donald, D. E., Lowensohn, H. S. and Pasyk, S. (1972). Coronary circulation in the conscious dog with cardiac neural ablation. *Circ Res, 31*, 129-144.

[40] Habecker, B. A., Gritman, K. R., Willison, B. D. and Van Winkle, D. M. (2005). Myocardial infarction stimulates galanin expression in cardiac sympathetic neurons. *Neuropeptides, 39*, 89-95.

[41] Haessler, R., Wolff, R. A., Chien, G. L., Davis, R. F. and Van Winkle, D. M. (1997). High spinal anesthesia does not alter experimental

myocardial infarction size or ischemic preconditioning. *J Cardiothorac Vasc Anesth, 11*, 72-79.

[42] Hardwick, J. C., Ryan, S. E., Beaumont, E., Ardell, J. L. and Southerland, E. M. (2014). Dynamic remodeling of the guinea pig intrinsic cardiac plexus induced by chronic myocardial infarction. *Auton Neurosci, 181*, 4-12.

[43] Hasan, W. (2013). Autonomic cardiac innervation: development and adult plasticity. *Organogenesis, 9*, 176-193.

[44] Hausenloy, D. J. and Yellon, D. M. (2008). Preconditioning and postconditioning: new strategies for cardioprotection. *Diabetes Obes Metab, 10*, 451-459.

[45] Hodgson, J. M., Cohen, M. D., Szentpetery, S. and Thames, M. D. (1989). Effects of regional alpha- and beta-blockade on resting and hyperemic coronary blood flow in conscious, unstressed humans. *Circulation, 79*, 797-809.

[46] Hopkins, D. A., MacDonald, S. E., Murphy, D. A. and Armour, J. A. (2000). Pathology of intrinsic cardiac neurons from ischemic human hearts. *Anat Rec, 259*, 424-436.

[47] Horackova, M., Armour, J. A. and Byczko, Z. (1999). Distribution of intrinsic cardiac neurons in whole-mount guinea pig atria identified by multiple neurochemical coding. A confocal microscope study. *Cell Tissue Res, 297*, 409-421.

[48] Huang, H. S., Pan, H. L., Stahl, G. L. and Longhurst, J. C. (1995). Ischemia- and reperfusion-sensitive cardiac sympathetic afferents: influence of H2O2 and hydroxyl radicals. *Am J Physiol (Heart Circ Physiol), 269*, H888-H901.

[49] Huang, M. H., Ardell, J. L., Hanna, B. D., Wolf, S. G. and Armour, J. A. (1993). Effects of transient coronary artery occlusion on canine intrinsic cardiac neuronal activity. *Integr Physiol Behav Sci, 28*, 5-21.

[50] Huang, M. H., Sylven, C., Horackova, M. and Armour, J. A. (1995). Ventricular sensory neurons in canine dorsal root ganglia: effects of adenosine and substance P. *Am J Physiol, 269*, R318-R324.

[51] Huang, M. H., Wolf, S. G. and Armour, J. A. (1994). Ventricular arrhythmias induced by chemically modified intrinsic cardiac neurones. *Cardiovasc Res, 28*, 636-642.

[52] Janes, R. D., Johnstone, D. E. and Armour, J. A. (1987). Functional integrity of intrinsic cardiac nerves located over an acute transmural myocardial infarction. *Can J Physiol Pharmacol, 65*, 64-69.

[53] Janig, W. (2014). Autonomic nervous system and inflammation. *Auton Neurosci, 182*, 1-3.

[54] Janig, W. (2014). Sympathetic nervous system and inflammation: a conceptual view. *Auton Neurosci, 182*, 4-14.

[55] Kaufmann, P. A., Rimoldi, O., Gnecchi-Ruscone, T., Bonser, R. S., Luscher, T. F. and Camici, P. G. (2004). Systemic inhibition of nitric oxide synthase unmasks neural constraint of maximal myocardial blood flow in humans. *Circulation, 110*, 1431-1436.

[56] Kawasaki, T., Azuma, A., Kuribayashi, T., Taniguchi, T., Asada, S., Kamitani, T., Kawasaki, S., Matsubara, H. and Sugihara, H. (2006). Enhanced vagal modulation and exercise induced ischaemia of the inferoposterior myocardium. *Heart, 92*, 325-330.

[57] Kember, G., Armour, J. A. and Zamir, M. (2013). Neural control hierarchy of the heart has not evolved to deal with myocardial ischemia. *Physiol Genomics, 45*, 638-644.

[58] Khalsa, S. S., Shahabi, L., Ajijola, O. A., Bystritsky, A., Naliboff, B. D. and Shivkumar, K. (2014). Synergistic application of cardiac sympathetic decentralization and comprehensive psychiatric treatment in the management of anxiety and electrical storm. *Front Integr Neurosci, 7*, 98.

[59] Kiernan, M. C., Walters, R. J., Andersen, K. V., Taube, D., Murray, N. M. and Bostock, H. (2002). Nerve excitability changes in chronic renal failure indicate membrane depolarization due to hyperkalaemia. *Brain, 125*, 1366-1378.

[60] Kimura, K., Ieda, M. and Fukuda, K. (2012). Development, maturation, and transdifferentiation of cardiac sympathetic nerves. *Circ Res, 110*, 325-336.

[61] Kingma, J. G., Jr. Armour, J. A. and Rouleau, J. R. (1994). Chemical modulation of *in situ* intrinsic cardiac neurones influences myocardial blood flow in the anaesthetised dog. *Cardiovasc Res, 28*, 1403-1406.

[62] Kingma, J. G., Simard, D., Voisine, P. and Rouleau, J. R. (2011). Role of the autonomic nervous system in cardioprotection by remote preconditioning in isoflurane-anaesthetized dogs. *Cardiovasc Res, 89*, 384-391.

[63] Kingma, J. G., Simard, D., Voisine, P. and Rouleau, J. R. (2013). Influence of cardiac decentralization on cardioprotection. *PLoS One, 8*, e79190.

[64] Krishnan, A. V. and Kiernan, M. C. (2009). Neurological complications of chronic kidney disease. *Nat Rev Neurol, 5*, 542-551.

[65] Kudej, R. K., Shen, Y. T., Peppas, A. P., Huang, C. H., Chen, W., Yan, L., Vatner, D. E. and Vatner, S. F. (2006). Obligatory role of cardiac nerves and alpha1-adrenergic receptors for the second window of ischemic preconditioning in conscious pigs. *Circ Res*, *99*, 1270-1276.

[66] Kuder, T. and Nowak, E. (2015). Autonomic cardiac nerves: literature review. *Folia Morphol (Warsz)*, *74*, 1-8.

[67] Kuder, T., Nowak, E., Szczurkowski, A. and Kuchinka, J. (2003). A comparative study on cardiac ganglia in midday gerbil, Egyptian spiny mouse, chinchilla laniger and pigeon. *Anat Histol Embryol*, *32*, 134-140.

[68] Lang, S. C., Elsasser, A., Scheler, C., Vetter, S., Tiefenbacher, C. P., Kubler, W., Katus, H. A. and Vogt, A. M. (2006). Myocardial preconditioning and remote renal preconditioning--identifying a protective factor using proteomic methods? *Basic Res Cardiol*, *101*, 149-158.

[69] Lavallee, M., Amano, J., Vatner, S. F., Manders, W. T., Randall, W. C. and Thomas, J. X. Jr. (1985). Adverse effects of chronic cardiac denervation in conscious dogs with myocardial ischemia. *Circ Res*, *57*, 383-392.

[70] Lefrandt, J. D., Smit, A. J., Zeebregts, C. J., Gans, R. O. and Hoogenberg, K. H. (2010). Autonomic dysfunction in diabetes: a consequence of cardiovascular damage. *Curr Diabetes Rev*, *6*, 348-358.

[71] Li, J., Xuan, W., Yan, R, Tropak, M. B., Jean-St-Michel, E., Liang, W., Gladstone, R., Backx, P. H., Kharbanda, R. K. and Redington, A. N. (2011). Remote preconditioning provides potent cardioprotection via PI3K/Akt activation and is associated with nuclear accumulation of beta-catenin. *Clin Sci (Lond)*, *120*, 451-462.

[72] Loukogeorgakis, S. P., Panagiotidou, A. T., Broadhead, M. W., Donald, A., Deanfield, J. E. and MacAllister, R. J. (2005). Remote ischemic preconditioning provides early and late protection against endothelial ischemia-reperfusion injury in humans: role of the autonomic nervous system. *J Am Coll Cardiol*, *46*, 450-456.

[73] Lujan, H. L., Palani, G., Zhang, L. and DiCarlo, S. E. (2010). Targeted ablation of cardiac sympathetic neurons reduces the susceptibility to ischemia-induced sustained ventricular tachycardia in conscious rats. *Am J Physiol Heart Circ Physiol*, *298*, H1330-H1339. doi:00955. 2009 [pii];10.1152/ajpheart.00955.2009 [doi].

[74] Mastitskaya, S., Marina, N., Gourine, A., Gilbey, M. P., Spyer, K. M., Teschemacher, A. G., Kasparov, S., Trapp, S., Ackland, G. L. and Gourine, A. V. (2012). Cardioprotection evoked by remote ischaemic

preconditioning is critically dependent on the activity of vagal pre-ganglionic neurones. *Cardiovasc Res*, *95*, 487-494.

[75] McAllen, R. M., Salo, L. M., Paton, J. F. and Pickering, A. E. (2011). Processing of central and reflex vagal drives by rat cardiac ganglion neurones: an intracellular analysis. *J Physiol*, *589*, 5801-5818.

[76] Minguet, G., Joris, J. and Lamy, M. (2007). Preconditioning and protection against ischaemia-reperfusion in non-cardiac organs: a place for volatile anaesthetics? *Eur J Anaesthesiol*, *24*, 733-745.

[77] Minisi, A. J. and Thames, M. D. (1991). Activation of cardiac sympathetic afferents during coronary occlusion: Evidence for reflex activation of sympathetic nervous system during transmural myocardial ischemia in the dog. *Circulation*, *84*, 357-367.

[78] Murphy, D. A., Thompson, G. W., Ardell, J. L., McCraty, R., Stevenson, R. S., Sangalang, V. E., Cardinal, R., Wilkinson, M., Craig, S., Smith, F. M., Kingma, J. G. Jr. and Armour, J. A. (2000). The heart reinnervates after transplantation. *Ann Thorac Surg*, *69*, 1769-1781.

[79] Murry, C. E., Jennings, R. B. and Reimer, K. A. (1986). Preconditioning with ischemia: a delay of lethal cell injury in ischemic myocardium. *Circulation*, *74*, 1124-1136.

[80] Nasr, N., Czosnyka, M., Arevalo, F., Hanaire, H., Guidolin, B. and Larrue, V. (2011). Autonomic neuropathy is associated with impairment of dynamic cerebral autoregulation in type 1 diabetes. *Auton Neurosci*, *160*, 59-63.

[81] Nathan, C. and Ding, A. (2010). Nonresolving inflammation. *Cell*, *140*, 871-882.

[82] Nguyen, B. L., Li, H., Fishbein, M. C., Lin, S. F., Gaudio, C., Chen, P. S. and Chen, L. S. (2012). Acute myocardial infarction induces bilateral stellate ganglia neural remodeling in rabbits. *Cardiovasc Pathol*, *21*, 143-148.

[83] Nielsen, V. K. (1974). The peripheral nerve function in chronic renal failure. 8. Recovery after renal transplantation. Clinical aspects. *Acta Med Scand*, *195*, 163-170.

[84] Oh, S. J., Clements, R. S., Jr. Lee, Y. W. and Diethelm, A. G. (1978). Rapid improvement in nerve conduction velocity following renal transplantation. *Ann Neurol*, *4*, 369-373.

[85] Ondicova, K. and Mravec, B. (2010). Multilevel interactions between the sympathetic and parasympathetic nervous systems: a minireview. *Endocr Regul*, *44*, 69-75.

[86] Pardini, B. J., Lund, D. D. and Schmid, P. G. (1989). Organization of the sympathetic postganglionic innervation of the rat heart. *J Auton Nerv Syst, 28*, 193-201.

[87] Pop-Busui, R. (2010). Cardiac autonomic neuropathy in diabetes: a clinical perspective. *Diabetes Care, 33*, 434-441.

[88] Przyklenk, K., Bauer, B., Ovize, M., Kloner, R. A. and Whittaker, P. (1993). Regional ischemic preconditioning protects remote virgin myocardium from subsequent coronary occlusion. *Circulation, 87*, 893-899.

[89] Przyklenk, K. and Kloner, R. A. (1998). Ischemic preconditioning: exploring the paradox. *Prog Cardiovasc Dis, 40*, 517-547.

[90] Qiu, Y., Tang, X. L., Park, S. W., Sun, J. Z., Kalya, A. and Bolli, R. (1997). The early and late phases of ischemic preconditioning. A comparative analysis of their effects on infarct size, myocardial stunning, and arrhythmias in conscious pigs undergoing a 40-minute coronary occlusion. *Circ Res, 80*, 730-742.

[91] Rajendran, P. S., Nakamura, K., Ajijola, O. A., Vaseghi, M., Armour, J. A., Ardell, J. L. and Shivkumar, K. (2016). Myocardial infarction induces structural and functional remodelling of the intrinsic cardiac nervous system. *J Physiol, 594*, 321-341.

[92] Randall, W. C., Kaye, M. P., Thomas, J. X. and Barber, M. J. (1980). Intrapericardial denervation of the heart. *J Surg Res, 29*, 101-109.

[93] Randall, W. C., Milosavljevic, M., Wurster, R. D., Geis, G. S. and Ardell, J. L. (1986). Selective vagal innervation of the heart. *Ann Clin Lab Sci, 16*, 198-208.

[94] Redington, K. L., Disenhouse, T., Strantzas, S. C., Gladstone, R., Wei, C., Tropak, M. B., Dai, X., Manlhiot, C., Li, J. and Redington, A. N. (2012). Remote cardioprotection by direct peripheral nerve stimulation and topical capsaicin is mediated by circulating humoral factors. *Basic Res Cardiol, 107*, 241.

[95] Rimoldi, O. E., Drake-Holland, A. J., Noble, M. I. and Camici, P. G. (2007). Basal and hyperaemic myocardial blood flow in regionally denervated canine hearts: an *in vivo* study with positron emission tomography. *Eur J Nucl Med Mol Imaging, 34*, 197-205.

[96] Rosengard-Barlund, M., Bernardi, L., Fagerudd, J., Mantysaari, M., Af Bjorkesten, C. G., Lindholm, H., Forsblom, C., Waden, J. and Groop, P. H. (2009). Early autonomic dysfunction in type 1 diabetes: a reversible disorder? *Diabetologia, 52*, 1164-1172.

[97] Rouleau, J. R., Simard, D., Rodrigue, N., Blouin, A. and Kingma, J. G. Jr. (2002). Myocardial blood flow after chronic cardiac decentralization in anesthetized dogs: effects of ACE-inhibition. *Auton Neurosci*, *97*, 12-18.

[98] Rubart, M. and Zipes, D. P. (2005). Mechanisms of sudden cardiac death. *J Clin Invest*, *115*, 2305-2315.

[99] Saraste, A., Ukkonen, H., Varis, A., Vasankari, T., Tunturi, S., Taittonen, M., Rautakorpi, P., Luotolahti, M., Airaksinen, K. E. and Knuuti, J. (2015). Effect of spinal cord stimulation on myocardial perfusion reserve in patients with refractory angina pectoris. *Eur Heart J Cardiovasc Imaging*, *16*, 449-455.

[100] Saxena, P., Newman, M. A., Shehatha, J. S., Redington, A. N. and Konstantinov, I. E. (2010). Remote ischemic conditioning: evolution of the concept, mechanisms, and clinical application. *J Card Surg*, *25*, 127-134.

[101] Serejo, F. C., Rodrigues, L. F., Jr. da Silva Tavares, K. C., de Carvalho, A. C. and Nascimento, J. H. (2007). Cardioprotective properties of humoral factors released from rat hearts subject to ischemic preconditioning. *J Cardiovasc Pharmacol*, *49*, 214-220.

[102] Singh, S., Johnson, P. I., Lee, R. E., Orfei, E., Lonchyna, V. A., Sullivan, H. J., Montoya, A., Tran, H., Wehrmacher, W. H. and Wurster, R. D. (1996). Topography of cardiac ganglia in the adult human heart. *J Thorac Cardiovasc Surg*, *112*, 943-953.

[103] Slavikova, J., Kuncova, J., Reischig, J. and Dvorakova, M. (2003). Catecholaminergic neurons in the rat intrinsic cardiac nervous system. *Neurochem Res*, *28*, 593-598.

[104] Sonoyama, K., Tajima, K., Fujiwara, R. and Kasai, T. (2000). Intravenous infusion of hexamethonium and atropine but not propranolol diminishes apolipoprotein A-IV gene expression in rat ileum. *J Nutr*, *130*, 637-641.

[105] Stevens, M. J., Dayanikli, F., Raffel, D. M., Allman, K. C., Sandford, T., Feldman, E. L., Wieland, D. M., Corbett, J. and Schwaiger, M. (1998). Scintigraphic assessment of regionalized defects in myocardial sympathetic innervation and blood flow regulation in diabetic patients with autonomic neuropathy. *J Am Coll Cardiol*, *31*, 1575-1584.

[106] Thompson, G. W., Horackova, M. and Armour, J. A. (1998). Sensitivity of canine intrinsic cardiac neurons to H2O2 and hydroxyl radical. *Am J Physiol*, *275*, H1434-H1440.

[107] Toombs, C. F., Wiltse, A. L. and Shebuski, R. J. (1993). Ischemic preconditioning fails to limit infarct size in reserpinized rabbit myocardium. Implication of norepinephrine release in the preconditioning effect. *Circulation, 88*, 2351-2358.

[108] Uchida, Y. and Murao, S. (1974). Excitation of afferent cardiac sympathetic nerve fibers during coronary occlusion. *Am J Physiol, 226*, 1094-1099.

[109] Vaseghi, M., Lellouche, N., Ritter, H., Fonarow, G. C., Patel, J. K., Moriguchi, J., Fishbein, M. C., Kobashigawa, J. A. and Shivkumar, K. (2009). Mode and mechanisms of death after orthotopic heart transplantation. *Heart Rhythm, 6*, 503-509.

[110] Vaseghi, M. and Shivkumar, K. (2008). The role of the autonomic nervous system in sudden cardiac death. *Prog Cardiovasc Dis, 50*, 404-419.

[111] Vergroesen, I., Merkus, D., Van Teeffelen, J. W. G. E., Dankelman, J., Spaan, J. A. E., Van Wezel, H. B., Noble, M. I. M. and Drake-Holland, A. J. (1999). Chronic cardiac denervation affects the speed of coronary vascular regulation. *Cardiovasc Res, 44*, 615-622.

[112] Wallis, D., Watson, A. H. and Mo, N. (1996). Cardiac neurones of autonomic ganglia. *Microsc Res Tech, 35*, 69-79.

[113] Weber, C. (2010). Far from the heart: Receptor cross-talk in remote conditioning. *Nat Med, 16*, 760-762.

[114] Weihe, E., Schutz, B., Hartschuh, W., Anlauf, M., Schafer, M. K. and Eiden, L. E. (2005). Coexpression of cholinergic and noradrenergic phenotypes in human and nonhuman autonomic nervous system. *J Comp Neurol, 492*, 370-379.

[115] Werner, R. A., Maya, Y., Rischpler, C., Javadi, M. S., Fukushima, K., Lapa, C., Herrmann, K. and Higuchi, T. (2015). Sympathetic nerve damage and restoration after ischemia-reperfusion injury as assessed by C-hydroxyephedrine. *Eur J Nucl Med Mol Imaging*.

[116] Yellon, D. M. and Downey, J. M. (2003). Preconditioning the myocardium: from cellular physiology to clinical cardiology. *Physiol Rev, 83*, 1113-1151.

In: Autonomic Nervous System (ANS)
Editor: Patrick Bernard Owens

ISBN: 978-1-63484-884-8
© 2016 Nova Science Publishers, Inc.

Chapter 2

VAGAL ACTIVITY ASCERTAINMENT FOR RISK ESTIMATION AND PROGNOSIS: WHAT IS EVIDENCE AND WHAT CAN BE SUPPOSED?

Thomas Kibbel, MD, PhD*

University Clinic Schleswig-Holstein, Campus Luebeck,
Medical Department I, Germany
LAFAA Laboratory for Contract Research in Clinical Pharmacology
and Pharmaceutical Analytics GmbH, Bad Schwartau, Germany

ABSTRACT

As is well known, the respective function of autonomic nervous system is at least partly responsible for anybody´s individual risk. In that concern it can be supposed by a series of investigations that the vagal part of autonomic function is more sensible reacting to noxious effects than the sympathetic one. Corresponding coherence is given by the more rapid recovery of sympathetic drive when autonomic function was formerly suppressed in general. Conversely, in time course of impairment as well when toxic effects will become stronger, the sympathetic response will become relatively more depressed than the parasympathetic one. This may explain that global parameters of heart rate variability (HRV), for example, sometimes had greater prognostic relevance than information

---

* Email: th.kibbel@gmx.de.

upon spectral analysis. As such, the ratio of special components may lead to inconsistent figures when valuation will be performed too much overall and without differentiation.

With respect to such complex coherences, additional hints are getting to more interest that particularly a reduced vagal function or the herewith furthermore reduced anti-inflammation and NO delivery should be responsible for a lot of complications. Such are elevating the risk for premature death. Therefore, one must be aware that beyond autonomic function in general especially vagal parts of autonomic nervous system should not be stressed unnecessarily. Anticholinergic effects without medical indication should be avoided if possible. On the other side it could be also demonstrated that the prognosis can be improved in several circumstances when vagal influences will become intentionally elevated. However, until now this was only found by electrical vagus nerve stimulation. Nevertheless, in this concern can be thoroughly assumed that the pharmacological potential should be promising as well, but surely more by the precondition that the respective aim corridor is known.

This hypothesis will be underlined if we look, for example, at the pleiotropic profile of (1) beta blockers, (2) statins and (3) metformin. All those agents is common (1) that they are reducing cardiovascular risks, (2) that they are reducing the incidence or severity of bacterial infections and (3) that they are also positively influencing cancer diseases regarding to lower incidence and progress. Consequently, (4) mortality was lower found in many studies even without further differentiation when these agents were given before. Furthermore is striking that in all three cases either the vagal activity in heart rate variability (HRV) analysis was found to increase or the sympathetic activity in muscle sympathetic nerve activity (MSNA) was found to decrease. Thus, one should really surprise that the aspect of functional alteration is not adequately taken into pharmacological consideration, especially if the safety of drugs or the advantage in comparison of drugs is concerned.

Likewise is not adequately realized that metformin, for example, is not only reducing the blood glucose and the mortality in general as well, but has furthermore positive effects (1) in different cancer diseases, (2) in different liver diseases, (3) in intestinal inflammation, (4) in rheumatoid arthritis and additionally (5) in diverse neurological diseases like Parkinson´s disease, multiple sclerosis, some forms of dementia, epilepsy and in ischemic stroke as well. (6) Furthermore, the risk of cognition decline was mostly reduced in diabetes. Regarding to autonomic function changes, today is already known that in most of patient groups mentioned above is typical that they are influenced by a diminished autonomic response, especially in the vagal determined part. And that all metformin effects should be exclusively referred to defined cell-biological or biochemical mechanisms is not even very probable. More unspecific influences should be also considered, surely at least as an environmental co-factor. Such can be improved by drugs but - more often - aggravated by drugs.

The existence of such unspecific but relevant effects will be underlined by the fact that, for example, any alcohol consume is elevating the incidence of infection and cancer, and the last, although invitro no increased cancerogenity was found until now. The coherences were only found and confirmed on the ground of retrospective observations. Furthermore is to consider that autonomic functions, for example, in diabetics and in patients with neurological diseases are typically changed similarly to alcohol dependent subjects. Analogously, elevated incidences of infection and cancer were often seen in such patient groups. Just inverse are the observational findings upon physical activity where specific molecular effects should be nearly excluded. Similar holds true for psychical stress, sleep deprivation, noise and air pollution. In this rather a sympathetic predominance or a lastly diminished oxygen supply should be more probable for etiology and pathogenesis.

For the assumption that more relevant unspecific effects may act on autonomic and immunologic level is also speaking that not only infections but also malignant diseases were more often ascertained (1) by the use of newer antidiabetics when are compared with metformin - as well as (2) when patients are receiving anesthesia or analgesia/sedation as well as (3) after application of erythrocyte concentrates. All could be well explained by a measurable reduction of autonomic/immunologic function.

On the ground of the above-discussed considerations the presented paper engaged on different aspects upon the autonomic modulation of physical functions and here especially on vagal parts. It is summarized (1) what is evidence from the literature, (2) what can be supposed by the existing data and (3) where may be potentials for practical use in the future. Accordingly, not only HRV analysis and MSNA are focused, moreover other non-invasive alternatives like pulse wave velocity, oxygen saturation or blood glucose variation are mentioned. On the other side diverse conflicting interests that are opposing against such investigations are nominated as well.

Keywords: autonomic nervous system, heart rate variability, vagal activity, all-cause mortality

WHAT IS KNOWN ABOUT THE CONNECTION OF AUTONOMIC FUNCTION AND PROGNOSIS?

There is growing evidence that status of autonomic function can be recorded non-invasively by several methods. At that, such ascertainment serves not only as a sign of physical fitness in healthy subjects, moreover, such ascertainment is of predictive importance when severely ill patients must be prognostically estimated. In this concern more and more results from the literature are reporting different influences on heart rate variability (HRV). The description of such phenomena is not really new. As such, in China already in the 3rd century A.D. was described that a too much regular heart beat rhythm is connected with increased probability of death [1]. This means that a variation of beat-to-beat interval is physiological, however, from this ectopic beats must be marked off because those must be viewed as unfavorable arrhythmic events.

Fundamentally the ascertainment is relatively simple and the arising costs can be even surveyed as well [2], for the collecting of relevant data can be performed on principle by everyone who is passably skillful [3]. Derivation of surface ECG is not a really problem when the rules of use are known. And the results in long-term can be transferred to a recorder, occasionally even wireless. Thus, the draft data set may be got by acceptable efforts. The following evaluation can be conducted by software systems that are available on the market. And an immediate medical assistance is not necessary under rest conditions.

The evaluated alterations of autonomic nervous system function can be validly and reliably detected already by the classic analysis of HRV [4]. Against this the also physiological circadian rhythm is to distinguish and the heart rate recovery after a defined physical or psychic burden as well. Such data are likewise important. But for giving estimation in a clear overview widely homogenous conditions must be present. Therefore the data in the literature are most often due to resting and supine or sitting position. This must be considered when interpreting the figures.

From the time course of RR interval length, respectively, from the heart beat number per time unit can be concluded that the heart rate at any moment is terminated by several influences; here is typical that they are acting in different special oscillations. All influences are cumulating to the punctual found heart rate [5, 6]. On the other side, because the partial effects are arriving the sinus node in different time spaces, we can conclude on the respective activities from the partial frequencies (e.g., sympathetic and vagal drive). This further means that if the central modulation is working more often the ability of the organism to adapt to special needs is much better. Therefore, a higher fluctuation rate serves as a sign of better health and more robustness [7, 8].

Furthermore, beyond the relevant reduction of HRV in absolute figures also the relation of the single compartments to each other is of importance. This is very relevant in determining the balance between sympathetic and parasympathetic power [4].

DEVELOPMENT OF PROGNOSTIC ESTIMATION IN THE PAST

In historical view was shown at first that the variability of RR intervals in the Holter ECG is relevant for prognosis after myocardial infarction. As such mortality was associated with global reduced heart rate variability [9-11]. Next was described that similar autonomic impairment can be used for declaring the complications in diabetes mellitus and in alcohol abuse as well [12-15]. Furthermore, estimation of depth of analgosedation was connected to a special reduction of HRV [16].

The derivation from level of sinus node indeed should lead to a specific alterations and mediately to typical relation of cardiovascular diseases. But there is a further link that a reduced HRV gives predictive hints upon the mortality probability that can be supposed overall [17, 18]. Thus, individually existing comorbidities as such as acute causes leading to death seem to have no more differentiating influence. Additionally, must be considered that in regions of better health services causes leading to death should be due to cardiovascular diseases only in about 37% [19]. Cancer diseases are at least second frequent in about 26%.

Hence, the assumption obtrudes that a depressed HRV should not only give information upon impending heart diseases or vascular diseases. Rather can be thoroughly supposed that the impaired autonomic function ascertained in the sinus node must not only restricted to the cardiovascular system but HRV reduction should be more interpreted as a sign of a central impairment of autonomic function in general. In the sense of this thesis only would be crucial that the individual modulation of autonomic function may be clear and differentiated measured by special influences on heart rate. However, the relevance should be more far-reaching for prognosis.

This further would also mean that a direct and therefore restrictive relation of long-term ECG and cardiovascular system should be abandoned. Associations of HRV with general autonomic function as such as with further severe diseases would become probable. Herein, regulation and repair mechanisms on cellular and molecular level should be involved too. Nevertheless, if a lot of disarrangements should be at least associated with the variation of heart rate sequence over time, we must be aware that such ascertainment may be rendered more difficult by arrhythmic events or artefacts. Such must be identified by valid mistake finding algorithms and must be eliminated before HRV calculation. For if not done, for example, ectopic beats, that must be negatively estimated, would be positively valued in the sense of physiological HRV.

Therefore, if following the thesis, as is described above, the autonomic state overall should present leading influences for development of diseases and complications. As such, the innate genetic preconditions [20, 21] would be additionally influenced by external factors like psychological stress [22, 23], air pollution [24, 25], food [26, 27], disturbance in day-night rhythm [28] and noise [29, 30]. This would further mean that impairments already by such causes and already occurred diseases may favor severe complications. And therapies may act in the same wrong direction, but perhaps may change to more normal figures and may so improve the situation in total.

In the concern of a more far-reaching importance of autonomic function, in the meantime can be estimated to be sure that the global parameters SDNN (time domain) and Total Power (frequency domain) in HRV analysis are mirroring the modulation overall. For differentiating the effects and influences the high-frequent parameters rMSSD (time domain) and HF Power (frequency domain) give information upon vagal parts of central modulation [4]. By contrast, measuring the sympathetic activity by HRV analysis is more difficult because the low-frequent (LF) Power is rather influenced by sympathetic drive; however, this compartment is additionally mixed by parasympathetic counterparts. Despite such difficulties evidence makes widely sure that the relation LF/HF as such as the LF-Power after normalization may sufficiently represent sympathetic activity. Apart from this is to consider that muscle sympathetic nerve activity (MSNA) as a direct method is surely superior to HRV for measuring the sympathetic drive [31, 32].

Overall is widely evident that the respective function of autonomic nervous system is at least partly responsible for anybody´s individual risk. As such, in distinctly ill subjects HRV figures are typically depressed over the whole spectrum of frequencies (very low frequency (VLF) Power until high frequency Power (HF) Power). Activations in absolute figures were only found in small size when more young and healthy persons were concerned and/or when situations after defined burden were valued.

However, to more clearing the situation must be differentiated what special impairment is more pronounced. Accordingly it can be supposed by a series of investigations that the vagal part of autonomic function is more sensible reacting to noxious effects than the sympathetic one. Therefore could be shown that changes in vagal function developed earlier than sympathetic parts and, hence, sympathetic parts are probably the leading factor in currently detecting of diseases [33-36]. Similar holds true for the more rapid recovery of sympathetic drive when autonomic function was formerly suppressed in general. Conversely, in time course of impairment as well when toxic effects will become more expressed the sympathetic response may be relatively more depressed than the parasympathetic one [37]. This may also explain that global parameters of heart rate variability (HRV) had sometimes greater prognostic relevance than information upon special spectral components, especially when evaluations will be performed too much overall and without differentiation.

The thesis of a widely non-specific phase dependent reduction of HRV will be underlined by several investigations. As such, an intravenous application of standardized endotoxin in one study was leading to a parasympathetic reduction [38] and in another study contrarily to a reduction especially of sympathetic parts [39]. By the conception that the parasympathetic modulation reacts more sensible on noxes and that diminishing of sympathetic activity takes place with delay, and then involvement leads increasingly to more decrease of sympathetic activity than to decrease of parasympathetic activity, the findings are not contradictory. For in the first study 0.5 ng/kg body weight was applied and in the second study 4 ng/kg body weight was applied. And in the concern of association of severity of infection the CRP correlated with HRV suppression [40, 41]. Simultaneously the development of septic shock was more associated with depression of sympathetic HRV compartments [42, 43]; likewise LF/HF ratio decreased increasingly to values of <1 [44, 45].

Similar was shown by elevated blood glucose levels in dependence of duration of diabetes mellitus. Whereas especially the vagus activity declined in the first phase of the disease [46-48], in the following more the sympathetic activity diminished and then was even the leading part [49, 50]. And such was not only remarkable in the concern of diagnose duration, the same was found in severe hyperglycemia in dependence of the individual elevated blood glucose. Until about 600 mg/dL a sympathetic predominance was typical and beyond of a parasympathetic predominance increases on the ground of further declining over the whole spectrum of HRV [37]. Herewith also the observation harmonizes that long-term expositions of polycyclic aromatic hydrocarbons were leading to HRV reductions in that the LF Power had the most prognostic value [51].

When taking together, overall can be surely suggested that in time course of impairment as well when toxic effects will become more expressed, the sympathetic response may become relatively more depressed than the parasympathetic one. And in consequence to this substantiated thesis in the recovery phase after doxepin or alcohol intoxication the LF Power part normalized more rapidly than the HF Power part [52-54]. Even such complex coherences may explain that global parameters of heart rate variability (HRV), for example, sometimes had greater prognostic relevance than information by spectral analysis. So, the ratio of special components may lead to inconsistent figures when valuation will be performed too much overall and without differentiation.

FOR WHAT PATIENTS AUTONOMIC ALTERATIONS ARE RELEVANT?

On the ground of sympathetic and parasympathetic nervous function is near at hand that severe degenerations like arrhythmias, hypertensive crises or acute heart failure can be well declared be respective alterations [55-57]. Accordingly was found that a reduced HRV, for example, is predictive for occurring of arrhythmias, in most cases when this is accompanied with a sympathetic predominance, but also in rather little cases when is accompanied by a parasympathetic predominance [58-61]. However, in other impairments like angina pectoris or endothelial dysfunction the explanation is not so simple. In this we have to consider that the effect of nitric oxide is clear connected with vagal activity [62-64]. And furthermore, from that evidence such publications must be distinguished in that not NO itself but NO donors were used [65-67]. Then often some contradictory was declared. As such, a reduction of vagal activity is reported. However, this opposite results can be well explained by different delivery mechanisms (redox processes) that cannot be avoided [68]. Nevertheless, endogenously generated NO itself correlates with vagal activity in a clear manner. Thus, upon that evidence can be expected that the vagal response also would have a central importance for early risk estimation.

Yet more patients can be conveyed to the vagal theory when one considers that the vagal function – afferent as well as efferent – is clear associated with the inhibition of proinflammatory functions [69]. And inflammatory processes as such as control mechanisms against are involved in many diseases. This also holds true for manifestation of malignancies [70-74], especially in the elderly [75] when vagal functions are typically reduced [76, 77]. By this the importance of central vagal activity in general is underlined [78-80]. The known coherences with NO and antiinflammation can be thoroughly explain the reported results [81-86]. Accordingly, also patients with different liver diseases [87], with intestinal inflammation [88], with rheumatoid arthritis [89] and additionally with diverse neurological diseases like Parkinson´s disease, multiple sclerosis, some forms of dementia, epilepsy and ischemic stroke have shown diminished parasympathetic activity [90-94]. And these are surely not all patient groups [95, 96].

Furthermore is noteworthy that (1) on the one hand the rapid HRV fluctuations are vagal, respectively, cholinergic determined, and (2) on the other hand was recently reported that the rapid gamma oscillations of the neuronal network can be artificially induced by acetylcholine [97]. A second precondition for development or sustaining of such effects was the sufficient supply of energy (glucose and oxygen). Lactate or pyruvate replacement decreased the amplitude even in high dosages (description of energy influences s. below).

Therefore, from the arguments mentioned above must be considered in the other direction that from changes in autonomic nervous system cannot be definitely and conclusively concluded on special diseases. However, from the figures in time course should be estimated how much the disease has proceeded and whether more severe complications must be expected or not. But the rather non-specific risk estimation should not be necessarily disadvantageous; for, so very much, what is connected with impairment and illness overall, will be focused to results of one measurement [98-105]. As such also was found that vagal activity correlates with cognitive capacity [106] and this should be further associated with mortality [107].

WHAT MAY UNDERLINE THE SPECIAL PROGNOSTIC RELEVANCE OF VAGAL ACTIVITY?

Although the causal coherences are not cleared until now, basically to results from the literature must be assumed that diminishment of vagal activity is an early sign of an inflammatory process which is prognostically disadvantageous for the patient independently from the origin [108, 109]. As such was found that HRV analysis in healthy non-smoking adults serves as an inflammatory indicator 4 years before the C-reactive protein will increase [110]. However, vagal activity is not only predictive in cardiovascular aspects but also in many other diseases [111]. This is even relevant for incidence and progress of malignant diseases [112-114]. Already a short overview gives hints that there is a common pathway that could lead to severe diseases, perhaps in accordance to individual preconditions.

This hypothesis will be underlined if we look, for example, at the pleiotropic profile of (1) beta blockers, (2) statins and (3) metformin. For all those agents is typical (1) that they are reducing cardiovascular risks [115-117], (2) that they are reducing the incidence or severity of bacterial infections [118-120] and (3) that they are also positively influencing cancer diseases regarding to lower incidence and progress [121-128]. Such influences may even act synergistically [129]. Consequently, (4) mortality was lower found in many studies even without further differentiation when these agents were given before. Furthermore is striking that in all three cases either the vagal activity in HRV analysis was found to increase or the sympathetic activity in muscle sympathetic nerve activity (MSNA) was found to decrease.

Similar positive alterations by figures of an increase of vagal activity, either absolutely or in relation to sympathetic activity, are described for omega-3 polyunsaturated fatty acids [130-132] and for vegetable polyphenols or flavonoids as well [133-137]. And also trimetazidine causes changes in sympatho-vagal balance in favor of vagal activity [138-140]. All agents are accompanied by positive clinical effects that are on principle the same that are described above as the pleiotropic effects. In accordance to that, the endothelin-1 level decreased and the NO level increased under trimetazidine [139]. Additionally, the anthracycline-induced cardiotoxicity was reduced by trimetazidine [141, 142].

Positive effects were also reported for acetyl salicylic acid and antioxidant agents, but such seem to be less expressed [143] and not always in the same extent in all patients [144]. Nevertheless, the more one is leaving the drugs that are on use, the less the investigations can be seen as finished. As such, positive effects on cancer and HRV are not only described for curcuminoids [145, 146] but also, for example, for green tea [147, 148]. And there is another more new topic that increasing bodyweight is associated with higher incidence of malignant diseases and furthermore with the following mortality [149-151]. Simultaneously, the LF/HF ratio in HRV analysis is more sympathetic influenced in obesity [152] and will reach rather normal levels when higher bodyweight will get to be reduced [153]. Furthermore in accordance, the LF/HF ratio was also reduced by not-excessive physical activity [154-156].

WHAT SHOULD BE CONCLUDED WHEN CONSIDERING THE WIDE PROFILE OF METFORMIN EFFECTS?

There is much evidence that statins but also β-blockers are exerting effects that were not standing in the field of vision when were studied first. However, this will be overtopped by the more wide potency of metformin. As such, metformin is not only reducing the blood glucose, but has positive effects on cardiovascular diseases and is reducing the mortality in general as well; furthermore the drug has likely positive effects (1) in different cancer diseases [126, 129, 157, 158], (2) in different liver diseases [159, 160], (3) in intestinal inflammation [126, 161], (4) in rheumatoid arthritis [162-164] and, additionally, (5) in diverse neurological diseases like Parkinson´s disease [165, 166], multiple sclerosis [167, 168], epilepsy [169] and in ischemic stroke as well [170, 171], but appearently only in chronic administration [172, 173]. (6) Similar holds true for reduction in risk of developing open-angle glaucoma [174] (7) and perhaps also with respect to protection of auditory hair cells [175]. (8) And extraordinarily, metformin improved ovarial blood flow and hormone profile in women with polycystic ovars [176, 177].

Furthermore, the risk of cognition decline should to be reduced by metformin in diabetes [178, 179] (9). However, there is a contrary result [180] that is discussed [181]. Upon this topic is published (1) that the biogenesis of Alzheimer´s amyloid peptides will be increased by metformin given as monotherapy [182], (2) that by an animal study this should be true in males but not in females [183]. By contrast, (3) increased incidence of dementia in type 2 diabetes was reduced by metformin, a little bit more than by sulfonylureas, and most when both drugs were given in combination [178]. This could possibly mean, that there is a dose relevant problem by metformin regarding to memory dysfunction. Furthermore, the differentiation of forms of dementia should be relevant. Benefits are especially described for vascular dementia [92].

Apart from the last discrepancies the questions arise at least, whether metformin is really a "super drug" and why effects have got to prominence that cannot be declared in first view. Latter could be widely unspecific [184-186] and could perhaps be also found elsewhere when one would merely further search consequently and accurately. Basically to the found and surely important improvement of vagal function, such can be thoroughly supposed.

Regarding to autonomic function changes today is already known that for most of the patient groups mentioned above is typical that they are influenced by a diminished autonomic response especially in the vagal determined part. And that all metformin effects should be exclusively referred to defined cell-biological or biochemical mechanisms like reduced induction by hypoxia-induced factor (HIF)-1α [187, 188], activation of AMP-activated protein kinase (AMPK) activating/reduction of mTOR signaling [189, 190], suppression of nuclear factor-kappaB (NF-κB) [191, 192] or decreased BACE1 protein expression [193] is not even very probable and should perhaps rather be re-questioned on principle [194-196]. Such was already mentionened in the concern of prostate cancer [197] and in the concern of stroke [198]. More unspecific influences like improvement of vagal activity or normalization of sympathovagal balance [199], even if perhaps only as a surrogate, should be considered, surely at least as an environmental co-factor. And such can be improved by drugs but - more often - also aggravated by drugs [200, 201].

Regarding to possible overall explanation there is more and more evidence that oxygen supply will become optimalized by metformin [202-204]. And energy dysfunction was shown to be most relevant for outcome in patients with severe head injury [205]. The existence of such unspecific but relevant effects must not be overlooked. Improvement by metformin was also noticed with respect of infection (10) [206, 207].

Nevertheless must not be ignored that a chronic kidney disease is a contraindication for metformin use according to the current guidelines [208]. This mainly, because metformin is renal eliminated and therefore an overdose is imminent. On the other side an improvement of HRV, especially of vagal parts, was advantageous in kidney diseases as well [209, 210]. As such is notified in the literature that the therapeutic benefit should perhaps overwhelm the risks if the agent would be given with caution [211]. Nevertheless, one must be aware that relative overdoses would lead to impairment of mitochondrial function [212]. And the question upon theoretical imaginable dose reduction or adequate dose adaptation is still open.

UNSPECIFIC ENVIRONMENT INFLUENCES: IS SUCH LEADING TO INITIATION OF INFECTION AND/OR CANCER?

The existence of unspecific but relevant effects even with respect of infection and cancer will be underlined by the fact that, for example, any alcohol consume is elevating the incidence or severity of infection [213, 214] and cancer [215], and the last, although invitro no increased cancerogenity was found until now [216]. Only the coexisting first metabolite and most toxic acetaldehyde was inciminated to be responsible for the risk in most reviews [217]. The coherences were only found and confirmed on the ground of retrospective observations. Furthermore is to consider that autonomic functions, for example, in diabetics and in patients with neurological diseases are typically changed similar to alcohol dependent subjects [90, 218-222]. Analogously, elevated incidences of infection and cancer were often seen in such patient groups. Just inverse are the observational findings upon physical activity where specific molecular effects should be nearly excluded [223]. Similar holds true for psychical stress, sleep deprivation, noise and air pollution. In this rather a sympathetic predominance or a lastly diminished oxygen supply should be more probable for etiology and pathogenesis.

As was mentioned above, changes in vagal function would develop earlier than sympathetic parts and, hence, the latter are probably the leading factor in currently detecting of diseases. This underpinned suppose is not in question on principle when, for example, the sympathetic response in sepsis and analgosedation will become more depressed than the parasympathetic one [39, 224]. Hereby must be recognized that vagal activity is absolutely also at a low level. And when additional negative influences will become present, such can the restricted capacity further worsen. Thus, a very impaired immune competence is to presume.

In that concern a recently occurred hospital epidemic of acitenobacter Baumannii should be remembered [225]. However, afterwards when the intensive care unit was closed and therefore no operations and, respectively, no ansthesia/analosedation had become necessary, no more new infections occurred. This observation in the concern of nosocomial infection can lead to the additional question, whether should perhaps not only be looked on frequency of hygiene procedures but also on anesthesia performance and regimes of analgosedation in the international comparison as well. And that a particular weakening of the organism can become relevant in the hospital and may be also involved in the epidemic was already supposed [225].

As such, a reduction of sedation depth [226] as well as a daily interruption has led to better outcome in actual investigations [227, 228], but rather not so in older studies overall [229]. Also in this issue the measurement of autonomic function should reveal some additional information. This should also be true in antibiotic use because was shown that antimicrobial agents are able to increase oxidative stress [230]; this further should diminish the protective vagal response [231, 232].

Similar can be surely supposed in the explanation of the observation that the application of erythrocyte concentrates has led not only to greater incidence of infections but also to greater incidence of malignant diseases [233, 234]. As a causal induction a redundant immunological challenge was hypothesized [234]. However, the observed complications were similar when autologous transfusions were compared with homologous ones. This is in accordance to other investigations that have not definitely shown that blood of patient´s own would lead to better outcome results [235, 236]. Hence, the destruction over time in both should be rather relevant because a late requirement of autologous material is not rational. In the conception overall that erythrocyte concentrates so would lead to an increased iron load, for exemple, negative influences on autonomic function cannot be excluded. As such, a reduction of LF und HF Power in HRV analysis was reported in thalassemia major and therapy [237]. In another study the LF/HF ratio correlated with the cardiac iron deposit [238], and such effects could be diminished by curcuminoids [239]. Furthermore, when looking on positive curcumin effects on cancer and HRV (s. above), an increased risk for infection and cancer in the sequence of erythrocyte substitution (especially the combination) cannot really surprise. In that concern is to remember that such complications occur more often in the elderly when autonomic functions, as is well known, are typically reduced. Similar serious events on the ground of reduced autonomic function and vagal depression (s. below) must be recognized in alcoholic [213, 215] and diabetic subjects [240-242].

ANTIDIABETICS AND ELEVATED INCIDENCE OF INFECTION AND CANCER

Beyond the connection of diabetes mellitus and greater numbers of infections and/or malignancies, moreover on the ground of sulfonylureas vs. metformin was fundamental shown that not only the disease for itself but also the used antidiabetics can be problematic [243]. In that concern in the last years was epidemiologically observed, that overall more bacterial infections and cancer manifestations must be expected under SGLT2 inhibitors and GLP-1 agonists [244-248]. As is described above, such might be possibly referred to a diminished vagal activity. However, by only a hypothesis until now, this should be confirmed or refuted by HRV measurement, and that not only in comparison to placebo but also in comparison to metformin as a third arm [248].

Only rudimentary and more or less industry associated investigations are published in open-access at which no guiding hint by HRV was found. However must be criticized that HRV figures were initial done or, perhaps, such were only published [249, 250]. Both results must be mirrored by independent fundamental results that were received by experimental investigations [251]. The fact, that different substance classes are concerned, is not really relevant on principle.

Beginning with the last published study [250], only brief 10-min segments after initial peripheral application were recorded in that study. Beyond of arterial stiffness and HRV in first time, advantageous lower blood pressure values were rendered to be prominent after 8-week empagliflozin use (however without presenting the concrete figures). This was pointed out as a sign of pleiotropy [250] whereas blood pressure decrease should be expected already by the action mechanism [252] (s. also blood pressure decreases in analogous agents [253]). Nevertheless, HRV values after an 8-week use were not given and, remarkably, not even the respective heart rates [250]. Similar is valid for canagliflozin [254]. Therefore, the strength of evidence should be rather low, and the long-term outcomes and safety are unclear [253].

When interpreting the data, one should consider on principle that not all alterations in the autonomic response must become perceptible in the initial phase. Rather a phase of central equilibration is to suppose [255], also when influences can be ascertained in early phase. For, in therapy course reflective tachycardia upon blood pressure decrease can occur on principle; so was seen by nifedipine [256] and was mentionend in the study on insulin and GLP-1

[249]. And when figures on heart rate were not given although may be thoroughly relevant [251] one must speculate that such figures were possibly not welcome in the industry sponsored study [250], and such effects in comparison to β-blockers, statins and metformin should rather be classified as "anti-pleiotrop."

Comparatively, not only increases of heart rate increases but also increases of blood pressure were seen by GLP-1 receptor stimulation [257, 258]. And such effects could be well explained by reduction of vagal activity if plasma levels of pancreatic peptide under GLP-1-infusion would be taken into consideration too [259, 260]. Furthermore was found that higher fasting plasma concentrations of GLP-1 should be positively associated with higher resting energy expenditure and negatively associated with respiratory quotient [260].

Further results on exendin-4 harmonize with a reduction of parasympathetic modulation. This GLP-1 agonist led to lower HRV figures overall (SDNN) [261] or to lower LF and HF Power that was referred to reduction of parasympathetic modulation [251]. Similar was published regarding to insulin or GLP-1 in less extent when more regional coherences were studied. As such, the first found correlation of insulin level to lower vagal activity disappeared after adjustment [249]. However, in clinical aspect the adjustment must not be relevant. Crucial is the resulting accumulative risk in practice. Risk assignment to single cofactors is not really of importance. In another study a parasympathetic reduction without level of significance was found [262]. And when central structures are definitely involved, the results were more unfavorable [251]. Not to neglect that such was already discussed [249]. Therefore, a direct comparison with metformin would surely bring more clearness. However, such was not done; only one direct comparison with metformin was published on vildagliptin and this only in one series of animal studies [263].

The results upon GLP-1 agonists could perhaps agree with the finding that these agents are elevating the insulin level and such was leading to a sympathetic amplification [264], but this only in insulin sensible subjects [265]. Overall the results are not consistent [266, 267]. As such, the authors of one industry sponsored study are hinting expressively at the end that their presented results were found by initial data, however, long-term investigation would be interesting [249]. Nevertheless, at least must be notified that in both relevant studies on SGLT2 inhibitors [250], respectively on GLP-1 agonists [249] no significant HRV alteration was found; by contrast under metformin vagal activity increased [199] or the LF/HF ratio decreased [268]. Already by this rough result a greater incidence of infection and cancer in comparison to metformin cannot surprise, and such can be detected in early phase of licensing process.

In another case the DPP-4 inhibitor vildaglitin was taken from the market in Germany because no agreement was obtained between the industry and the care providers. And this although the HRV results were not even unfavorable [263, 269, 270]; however, the above described method is not adequately used for comparison as a standard. Furthermore, cognitive faculties should be less impaired under DPP-4 inhibitors [271]. However, comparative studies to standard of metformin are not required although it cannot be excluded that guiding information will be got by low size of patients per subgroup [90, 255, 272, 273], when the investigation result is open and when the investigation is proper planned. Patient numbers of 10.000 and more [274, 275] should perhaps even not be necessary at first and only indicated for confirmation of the preliminary but hinting results (perhaps also for their refutation). Furthermore we can expect that information already during phase-1 studies would be got that would help to avoid later withdrawal from the market. So, ineffective costs may be minimized (but the sales until the recall as well). And concerning to first-in-man studies themselves can be supposed that severe adverse events should be detected more early when experiences on typical figures of autonomic function depression are present.

However, this also would mean that the usually practice of ascertaining the safety of drugs in contrast to placebo on top would neglecting the aspect on principle, that additional positive pleiotropic effects which have been proven in standard therapies are not requested [276]. As such, with respect to survival overall by empagliflozin, patients with acute coronary syndrome, with stroke as well as with cancer were excluded in the safety evaluation [277], although clear positive effects in that concern were found by metformin (s. above). In another case an underlined increasing of pneumonia/sepsis was perhaps not adequately pursued by the competent institutions [278]. On the other side in a series of SGLT2 inhibitors the FDA warned of diabetic ketoacidosis development [279] that is often triggered by infections [280] and in that HRV is typically strong depressed [37]. And under the GLP-1 agonist lixisetanide already in placebo comparison indeed no increased risk of cardiovascular complications was seen but also no respective decreased risk [281]. Remarkably, this agent is no more availably in Germany in the meantime.

ALTERATIONS OF AUTONOMIC FUNCTION IN PARKINSON'S DISEASE

HRV alterations increasingly take part in the graduation of neurological diseases whereas one should await even the first results on altered autonomic nervous function from neurology [282]. As such, respective impairment was found in Parkinson's disease. Especially vagal activity was concerned [283], and that in dependence from duration after diagnosis [90, 220], and more at night [284] or at sleep [285]. By considering these coherences the higher incidence of infection cannot really surprise [286]. Also the detected courses of death overall can be well explained by the restricted autonomic function [287]. This assumption is further underlined by a longer duration of QTc interval [288, 289].

And in the concern of association of Morbus Parkinson with cancer diseases in the higher developed countries rather an inverse relationship was seen [290] if single reports in the other direction are neglected [291, 292]. However, by contrast a positive association was ascertained in Eastern Asia [293]. Transferred to the consideration mentioned above, other results have shown that ergot-derived dopamine agonists would exert a sympathetic predominance (LF nu increase and HFnu decrease in supine position) [294] as well as a higher incidence of cancer [295]. By contrast, HRV overall increased by the use of levodopa [296, 297]. Furthermore was also suggested that the centrally derived respiration will be normalized [298]. Accordingly, occurrence of malign melanoma was independent from the use of levodopa [299]. And ergot derivates like bromocriptine are playing only a minor role at least in Europe and Northern America [300], but not so in Eastern Asia [301, 302]. Therefore the results overall agreed with the respective cancer incidence. The vagal competence should here also be guiding.

AUTONOMIC DYSFUNCTION IN MALIGNANCIES AND OUTCOME

On the ground of the alcoholic effect profile repeatedly was pointed to autonomic alterations. Typical is a general impairment and a development of sympathetic predominance. Herewith harmonize the figure of the "Holiday Heart syndrome" in early withdrawal [53] and the state in dependent persons as well [12-13]. Similar changes were seen by moderately elevated blood glucose levels [303] and in diabetes mellitus in the initial phase [304]. And in inflammatory diseases of the gut also an impairment of autonomic function especially of the vagal part must be supposed [305]. And, remarkably, an increased incidence of malignant diseases was observed in all these predispositions [241, 242, 306, 307].

First connections of HRV with cancer are basing on investigations of 2010. In those the authors found that a more diminished HRV should be associated with shorter survival. But in detailed interpretation only the SDNN as a global parameter was of predictive importance [308, 309] and, moreover, the heart rate itself should perhaps more suitable for estimation [310]. However, this seeming incapacity cannot surprise. All tumor entities to estimate in one direction and additionally to overlook different classes of drugs, especially the opioids, do not really make sense. Thus, no clear dependencies upon vagal suppression should be expected; for better knowledge differentiated evaluations must be performed.

Accordingly to breast cancer recently could be shown that special alteration of autonomic nervous function on the vagal side is connected to breast cancer [114, 311]. Therefore, a monitoring by HRV was explicitly suggested. Further could be found that physical activity would lead on the one hand to improvement of vagal function and on the other side was associated with better prognosis. Similar holds true for other non-lung cancers [312]. As such we have to consider that reduction of vagal activity is not only relevant in cardiovascular diseases [313] but also beyond [74, 111]. However, the sympathetic predominance before development should be more relevant in solid tumors, i.e., in tumors that are representing the greater size [314]. Thus, a statement in general is not adequate. This is underlined, for example, by the findings that carbachol and pirenzepin strengthened the growth of experimental induced prostate cancer [315]. And vagal response was shown to be increased by acutely given pirenzepin [316]. Remarkably, prostate cancer should be less connected to alcohol abuse [317] whereby vagal reduction is typical [318, 319].

Similar should be true in blood based cancers [314]. So is to conclude that a confirmation is needed in what extent the connections that were epidemiologically found by a broad data set are really relevant for the individual sub-form of cancer. Nevertheless should be sure that the autonomic nervous system is involved in tumor manifestation and tumor growth [320-322]. As such is already pointed out that cellular repair mechanisms should work better when vagal nerve activity is intact and when sympathetic nerve activity is not overstimulated [314]. This may underline that also an impairment on functional level should influence the immunologic response and therefore should favor cancer manifestation in special circumstances. By the conception that wrong cell structures or metabolism products are not eliminated in adequate extent, a greater cancer incidence can be thoroughly explained by defined expositions and in older age as well [75-77].

HOW CAN THE EFFECTS ON MALIGNANCIES BY VAGAL ACTIVITY BE DECLARED?

Already in the first half of the 20th century Otto Warburg had described that for tumor tissues is typical that energy would be generated by glycolysis although evidently no absolute oxygen deficit exists. Accordingly, this rather disadvantageous way for energy generation is called "Warburg effect" or "aerobic glycolysis" although this means a contradiction by itself. The way is unfavorable because only 2 Mol ATP/glucose are generated by glycolysis and 36 Mol ATP/glucose are generated by mitochondrial oxidative phosphorylation [323, 324]. However, hereby is not realized that intermediately originated lactate [325, 326] can also be used for energy supply by oxidation [327, 328] as was described for central compartments [97, 329]. The question is open until now in what extent this way is used and how much this is dependent from the regional oxygen concentration. Only was widely disproved that tumor tissues should be exclusively able to win their energy by glycolysis [323]. In this concern must be considered that no energy can be got without oxygen and that the oxygen demand in the CNS is 10fold higher than in the periphery [97]. Furthermore was shown that physical training leads to increased oxygen consumption [330]. This correlates with better HRV.

Thus, at first the question arises how all the findings can be concluded to a consistent hypothesis. As such is evident that two metabolic pathway exist for ATP production. First is oxidative phosphorylation under aerobic conditions and second is glycolysis under anaerobic conditions. Both possibilities exist parallel to each other on principle; however, glycolysis plays no relevant role when oxygen supply is high. However, if oxygen is decreasing glycolysis becomes more and more important ("Pasteur effect") [331] and so the substrate becomes very poor in glucose [332, 333]. Such increased consumption rate in tumor diseases could be verified by positron emission tomography already in 1987 [334]. Simultaneously by this hypothesis the concentration of lactate would increase in great extent [335]. However, such effect should be only of intermediate relevance because lactate itself may be oxidatively metabolized with precedence already on the ground of high mass effect and furthermore via monocarboxylate transporter (MCT)-1 [327, 336]. Similar coherences were supposed in septic patients by fentanyl use [224]. However, although this development may be plausible, it is not proven. The Warburg effect is still in discussion [324, 337].

Further is known that a diminished oxygen supply acts negatively on the autonomic functions already in healthy subjects. Accordingly, a deficit of oxygen will produce reactions that preserve the organism against tissue hypoxia. In that frame the initiated cascade leads to adaptations in the cardiovascular system too. Especially prominent is the hypoxia-caused sympathetic activation and, perhaps rather, the respective parasympathetic deactivation what can be at first ascertained by heart rate increase, by blood pressure increase and/or by increase of heart-time-volume [338]. Such alterations can be transferred to an objective level, e.g., by HRV analysis [339, 340]. Hence, on this base the relative sympathetic response increased during acute exposure to hypoxia and the parasympathetic response decreased not only in relation to sympathetic influences but also in absolute figures [341, 342]. Additionally in hypoxia was found that the parasympathetic reactivation ascertained by heart rate recovery was prolonged after submaximal exercise [343]. With respect to general encephalopathy [344], hypoxia was also connected with development of low blood glucose concentrations [345, 346]. This may even declare the currently discussed hypoglycemia under tramadol [347, 348], and perhaps also that under methadone [349, 350].

All the descriptions would be consistent, if one postulates additionally that the oxygen supply should be reduced in the tumor tissue because of diminished perfusion. By the conception that the O_2 supply is relevantly reduced in the last widow [351], one can suppose that the availability will increase under nitric oxide. For this is speaking that the NO level correlates positively with HF Power of HRV and therefore with vagal activity [340]. From this may be concluded that also the energy supply should be improved in the malignant and in the healthy tissue as well. In the case that energy is not enough available, on the one hand the malignant and perhaps even more robust tissue will be impaired; on the other side it could be that the healthy and perhaps less robust tissue will be also impaired. So, the intention of lowering the oxygen supply is possibly not leading to aim in humans.

By increase of oxygen both tissues will be better provided with energy [352]. This perhaps would favor the cancer growth. Therefore a simultaneously conduction of specific chemo- or radiotherapy should be right;

a respective combination therapy is described as to be advantageous [353-357]. An increase of oxygen by better perfusion would harmonize with a vagal improvement as well as with an improved NO effect [62-64]. Positive effects can be expected if not only the O_2 supply will be elevated but also if the tumor will be attacked by specific therapy [354, 358]. Nevertheless, positive as such as negative netto-effects by NO are not mutual excluding [359, 360]. As such, a better perfusion, e.g., by giving simvastatin led to better response of chemotherapy [361, 362] and of X-ray radiotherapy as well [363]. On the other side metformin had no positive effect in cytostasis by itself; however, when giving in combination with doxorubicin tumors were weped out and remission was prevented [364].

HOW TUMOR CACHEXIA AND AUTONOMIC IMPAIRMENT COULD BE CONNECTED?

Inflammatory processes are also strongly involved in tumor cachexia [365] that can be influenced by physical activity [366, 367]. This should be most important for space of survival [368]. In association to hypothesis mentioned above, perfusion would by insufficient as well and therefore the energy supply in the tumor tissue would not be adequate. The O_2 deficit would be in accordance to the likewise assumed lactate shuttle via monocarboxylate transporter (MCT)-1 [327, 369]. Simultaneously quasi a steal effect would become present that leads to shortage and wasting in the whole organism [370]. Under this conception the glucose expenditure should be monitored [371].

Furthermore, by increasing NO effects or by increasing parasympathetic activity can be declared why giving of omega-3 polyunsaturated fatty acids [130-132] will improve energy supply and more survival as well [372, 373]. This would mean that further substances that are increasing vagal competence should have similar positive effects in the course of disease. Concerning to positive influences by megestrol acetate, medroxyprogesterone and ghrelin [374] is published regarding to the two last agents that they would increase vagal parts of HRV and they would decrease sympathetic parts of HRV [375-378]. Beyond of, not only figures of HRV were improved but also the respiration under Medroxyprogesterone [379]. Upon megestrol acetate none is published. As such, the HRV results that were actually ascertained on cardiovascular questions harmonize very well with an increased strength of antiinflammation and tissue perfusion as well. Thus, also chocolate should exert positive effects on tumor cachexia [133, 134]. However, such overall is only speculative until now, whenever the cumulation of plausibility is striking. Not to ignore is that vagal activity had also decreased in ischemic stroke [79, 80]. And in therapy course an increasing of vagal activity was advantageous for prognosis.

ASPECTS CONCERNING DICHLOROACETATE

The preliminary results on dichloroacetate are promising as well. Although the investigations were not finished, rather nonspecific influences like vagal activity, antiinflammation and NO effects should also be involved in the spectrum of mechanism [380]. Accordingly, investigations have shown that dichloroacetate should strengthen the oxidative metabolism and should diminish glycolysis [356]. This was associated with effects like increasing of apoptosis and reducing of hypoxia-inducible factor (HIF)-1α [381]. This could lead to the assumption that similar basics are perhaps responsible for the reduction of tumor growth and angiogenesis [382].

CAN VAGAL THEORY BE TRANSFERRED TO THE ASSOCIATION OF MEAT CONSUME AND CANCER?

On the ground of above described coherences the question arises, whether the recently mentioned increase of cancer incidence induced by meat consume [383, 384] could perhaps be nearer declared. Upon epidemiologic data the WHO attributed processed meat as "cancinogen (group 1)" and red meat as "probable carcinogen (group 2A)" [385]. However, the question regarding to causality is open. By the idea that every human can only satiate once, a greater consumption of red meat or processed meat would imperatively lead to displacement of vegetables and fish. Further was found that food of plant origin is more often associated with protective effects against inflammation [386-389]. And prevention by fish oil was manifold proven [390, 391]. However by the width of confidence interval [392] can be also concluded that the number of co-factors should be large.

Nevertheless is not clear in detail why the meat consumption had led to the found negative effects. Incriminated are nitrite and heme iron [393], advanced glycation products [394], but also polycyclic aromatic hydrocarbons, heterocyclic amins, N-nitroso compounds and macromolecular oxidation products [395]. Nevertheless, greater consumption of red meat and greater consumption of processed meat have led to unfavorable concentrations of inflammatory biomarkers [383, 396, 397]. Therefore, on the ground of considerations mentioned above can thoroughly be expected that the risks can be nearer specified when measuring changes in autonomic regulation. However, for estimation the risk in adequate extent, we have to consider that the numbers of attributes deaths were 12fold higher by smoking, 7,5fold higher by alcohol use and 2,5fold higher by air pollution [398]. Here are the greater potencies for prevention. Nevertheless is conspicuous that observed complications by red meat consumption were fairly similar to that were seen by giving erythrocyte concentrates (s. above). And considering that several relevant triggers should be absorbed, the parallels must not surprise.

For completing the complex field cognition in association to vagal activity [106] was worse under meat consumption [399] and, by contrast, was better under chocolate consumption [400]. The latter is in accordance to the expected connection too [133,134].

CHANGES OF AUTONOMIC FUNCTION FOR EXAMINATION OF ILLNESS AND THERAPY IN TIME COURSE

Already the descriptions until here should lead to the founded hypothesis that illnesses, as such as drug therapies in time course, can be better and, more than all, currently estimated by co-considering of autonomic alterations. As such was shown in breadth that particularly the vagal activity is of importance. And when considering that many drugs have anticholinergic side effects, more justification for such investigation is not necessary. Nevertheless, the number of anticholinergics is much higher [401] than the number of that are favoring vagal responses. Accordingly was often shown that the parameters in HRV analysis that are representing vagal activity would be influenced by a lot of drugs generally [256, 296, 297, 402-406] and by oncologic agents especially [74, 407-410]; beyond of, also radiotherapy may decrease vagal activity more than sympathetic activity [411].

In this concern was further shown that dexamethasone may improve not only the vagal function [405] but also the gas exchange [412]. This is in consistence with the results that were found in induced hypoxia [341, 342]. Also NO concentration became higher in fibroblasts under dichloroacetate

[413] and the cytostatic effect of cisplatin increased as well [414]. A similar synergistic effect was ascertained under metformin/cisplatin [415]. And hypoxia via HIF-1α is considered to be responsible for transactivation of genes and accumulation of metabolites that promote tumor growth and metastasis [416].

Hence, sufficient monitoring is most important already in metformin use [276] and especially in high risk subjects [417-420]. However this aspect is not adequately taken into consideration until now. For, by this way the response of conducted therapy [410, 421] as such as the risks of therapy can be early estimated. Likewise could be acknowledged whether a change of therapy should be preferred. So it should not really surprise when the results of special regimes grounding on 5-year survival rates may be possibly obtained much earlier.

On the other side we are not allowed to neglect that agents, that are exerting rather advantage effects overall, may be overdosed as well. This can be dangerous for the patient in similar extent. So, difficulties are arising already in practice because clinicans do not know until now what aim should be aspired to achieve best outcome. Although the retrospective evaluation of changes by special conditions is indeed necessary at first on principle, nevertheless this is quite simple. Unequal more difficult is therapy steering because one must know what aim value, respectively rather, what aim corridor is optimal for the individual patient.

Accordingly, broad inquiries must be performed at first because overdoses or even to hasty applications may lead to complications as well [421]. As was shown for blood glucose levels, to high but also to low concentrations may lead to diminished autonomic function [37, 422, 423]. And that there should optimal ranges exist for the patients is underlined by the comparison of thyroid hormone deficieny vs. subclinical hyperthyroidism. Higher LF/HF ratios as signs of blunted vagal response were seen in both conditions [424, 425]. This holds true also when drug combinations are concerned. As such, an unexpected death in accordance to vagal predominance was seen under fingolimod und lorsatan [426].

HRV MONITORING OF FINGOLIMOD IN MULTIPLE SCLEROSIS FOR EXAMPLE

Investigations on relapsing-remitting multiple sclerosis have shown that vagus activity is reduced when patients are not treated [427-429] and that the deficit can be substituted by sphingosine 1-phosphate receptor modulators like fingolimod [421]. From the decription of typical complications in the initial phase of therapy [430, 431] one may imagine that such side effects should be widely similar to relative overdoses of metformin [432]. Likewise, initial fingolimod led to bradycardia, to intermittent AV block, to paroxysmal atrial fibrillation and to vagal increase when HRV analysis was performed [421, 433, 434]. Remarkably, in association of vagal activity with cancer reduction was further found that fingolimod (FTY720) was acting against liver tumor metastasis [435, 436]. Taking together, some authors have stated that fingolimod therapy may probably be monitored by HRV analysis, also because regulation during therapy course developed to more sympathetically influenced modulations [437]. Therefore, a broad field of HRV application is suggested [438].

Also investigations to further sphingosine 1-phoasphate receptor modulators are interesting [439]. Best is known on ponesimod. In this (1) compatibility and safety were comparable to fingolimod [440] and (2) the side effects are increasing in dependence from higher dosage [441]. In detail are described i.a. bradycardias, and in another study also block figures [442]. However, such effects were disappearing again in the course of therapy [443, 444]. Part of authors were wondering about [441], however it must be remarked that no alterations according to autonomic function were recorded.

WHICH CURRENT OPEN QUESTIONS SHOULD BE OBVIOUSLY REVISIONED ON AUTONOMIC FUNCTION?

Apart from the current discussion about effects by meat, fish and vegetable/fruit consumption on cancer (s. above) further question must arise, especially when the use of sugar vs. sugar exchange substances vs. saccharines is concerned. And concerning to potato consumption [399] is interesting how acrylamide in fried potato products is not only increasing the CRP [445] but is also impairing the autonomic function and so may perhaps favor some cancers [446]. Seen overall, regarding to cancer incidence in dependence of foodstuffs as good as nothing is known [447-449].

Even when not forestalling the final valuation, dimethyl fumarate should rather be connected with more or less unspecific effects [450-456]. However, there is also a report about a specific participation of hydroxycarboxylic acid (HCA)-2 receptors in therapy of multiple sclerosis [457]. Nethertheless, several publications exist that are describing positive dimethyl fumarate influences in malignant diseases [458, 459], not to speak of similar positive effects in psoriasis [460]. Thus, the question is very interesting how eventual changes in autonomic function are present behind.

In Morbus Alzheimer the sympathetic functions surely are more reduced [90, 93]; however, in another study vagal activity was also reduced in response to tilting [461]. Apart from alteration in the disease itself, repeatedly was found that vagal function will be (perhaps additionally) reduced by central cholinesterase inhibitors [462-464]. However, in another investigation such was only seen in initial phase; by long-term use an increase of vagal activity was found [255]. Unfortunately, the discrepancies upon direct effect vs. feed back vs. adaptation are not clearly resolved by continuous data until now. Therefore also the questions on cardiac autonomic control in close concern and on potentially further vagal influences are not finally answered. The published data to benefits by donepezil [465-467] are not always in accordance with the changes of autonomic function [468, 469]. Likewise, positive local effects by rivastigmin are not able to conclude on possible central changes in general [470].

However, not only valuations on drug therapy and on food influences can be acquired, furthermore statements on toxicology by agents can be achieved that are in the current discussion. As such, nearer information could perhaps be got. For example, carcinogenic potency of herbicides like glyphosate [471, 472] should be better classified whatever the direction is [473]. If the relevant effects could be currently achieved by measuring autonomic function, one must not wait until the figures on mortality can be retrospectively calculated. Although from the literature more vagal effects can be expected by glyphosate [474], however, such can be also risky for farmers and consumers when possible analogies to fingolimod overdoses [421, 433, 434] and to metformin overdoses [432, 475] are considered.

One special look should also be done on antibiotics because they may increase oxidative stress in general [230] and probably more by ones than by others [476]. This would further decrease vagal activity [477], and in the sequel the liability to nosocomial re-infection will also increase [478-480]. Hereby a phase dependency can be supposed [481] because in the course of infection and sepsis the sympathetic impairment should become more and more relevant. Vagal deficiency will be overtopped by sympathetic deficiency. Hence, in severe sepsis and septic shock LF/HF ratios of <1 in HRV are typical [42-45]. Such development can be already expected on the ground of different endotoxin exposure [38, 39]. And such will additionally increase under alcohol abuse [214]. The leading cause should be the dysfunctional gut barrier; but bacterial overgrowth as such as delayed endotoxin clearence cannot be excluded on principle [482].

And this enumeration surely mentioned not all relevant influences. Also environment factors like noise and air pollution [483, 484] or psychic stress can depress the vagal response and so may impair the connected regulations [485]. And regarding to air pollution also deleterious effects by mercury emissions from coal-fired power plants [486] should be probably detected by HRV analysis, if such is relevant [487, 488].

However should be assumed that not all impairments of HRV can be estimated to be equal when were of different origin. By contrast, also is not probable that effects in the same direction in multimorbidity would not increase the risk overall. Additive effects like QTc prolongation by drugs are likely. But contrariwise can be expected that an unfavorable autonomic level is reversible on principle. And this not only by electric stimulation [81, 82] but also pharmacologically what already the effect profil of metformin is hinting.

WHICH CONCRETE PROGRESS CAN BE EXPECTED BY MEASUREMENT OF AUTONOMIC FUNCTION?

Apart from environment and probably from food effects can be thorougly supposed that more comprehensive drug profiles can be achieved by analysis of autonomic state. On principle, this concerns all agents as were listed, for example, in the priscus list for elderly subjects [489]. By knowing single effects of any drug physicians and pharmacists should be able to conclude on probable effects in total. Fundamentally can be expected that pharmacotherapy can be individually adjusted and optimalized. Drug interactions and incompatibilities should be mirrored by decreases in autonomic function. Also relative overdoses and underdoses should be detected.

However, if dosage is supposed to be too high or too low, the dosis cannot be changed at pleasure already from law aspects. And discontuniation is not the resolution in every case. Only by the aid of additional monitoring procedures may be justified that doses should be modified. Accordingly a extended online ECG as diagnostic tool could be helpful. Simultaneously can be probably ascertained whether, for example, an antidiabetic or oncologic therapy should be successful or not. A response of conducted therapy could be recognized when typical autonomic alterations are developing or not [306,

421]. Therefore, it can be extected that an extensive and current therapy monitoring should be available by an extended analysis of usually conducted Holter ECG and by that the outcome will be improved overall [490, 491]. Beyond of, an additional level will be introduced that demasks analogies and intersections and so would lead to better understanding of connections.

In that concern was shown, for example, that statins are able to reduce the intraocular pressure [492]. So was further found that statins would prevent against open angle glaucoma [493]. Similar was achieved by physical activity [494, 495]. Both interventions are common that sympathovagal balance will be normalized [496-500].

Moreover is reported that more patients receiving statins and suffering muscle symptomes were typically rather physically active [501] and therefore a comparable predominance of vagal function should be present. This can lead to the supposition that a relative overdose of statins could be perhaps diagnosed by analysis of autonomic function. On the other side cardiovascular advantages by statins are especially mentioned for patients that are typically influenced by a sympathetic predominance and/or in that an overall less autonomic adaptation competence can be assumed (1. patients with manifest atherosclerotic vascular disease, 2. with LDL-C >190 mg/dL, 3. with diabetes mellitus and LDL-C >70 mg/dL and 4. with global 10-year risk for developing of a atherosclerotic vascular disease >7,5% and LDL-C >70mg/dL [13, 502-505]).

And according to acute ischemic stroke was found that statin use may improve outcome when patients were treated before [506]. Here must be considered that ischemic stroke is associated with impairment of HRV [507], with QT prolongation [508] and with increased QT dispersion as well [509]. Remarkably, all parameters will be improved by statins [510, 511].

Hereby may be well supposed that extended data from ECG should surely reveal informations even beyond the usual boundary of physician specialization. Interconnections can complete the figure of multimorbidity (e.g., cardiovascular complications in several neurologiocal disorders [221, 512-516]; similar surely holds true fore cardiovascular disease and normal-tension glaucoma [517, 518], respectively for open-angle glaucoma [519, 520]). Another example is the higher UV sensitivity of males that had led to greater incidence of skin cancer in experimental studies [521, 522]. With respect to proinflammatory/anti-inflammatory involvement is consistent that vagal activity in premenopausal women is higher than in respective men, at least in relation to sympathetic activity [76, 77]. Similarly, the incidence of severe bacterial infection was higher in such men than in such women [523,

524]. This can also be explained by higher LF/HF ratio in men [525]. This short item list may declare how the HRV analysis should contribute to understanding of observations.

However, such associations cannot be only declared by receptor stimulation and special signaling. More unspecific influences like improvement of vagal activity or normalization of sympathovagal balance [199] are likely, at least as an environmental co-factor. Remarkably, even this individual and current state is at least part of prognostic relevance. By online measuring the autonomic state in detail, vital risks can be estimated simultaneously and currently. And such is also dependent from therapy. Hence, in relation to special groups, mortality that is to expect cannot only be ascertained much earlier, rather more, risks can be estimated when patients are still alive and not when have died in part. This would further mean that survival/nonsurvival rates as dichotomy criterion could be transferred to a continuous variable that can be even influenced and is at least reversible in part. 5-year survival rates, perhaps, may only confirm premature results when the method will have been validated.

Moreover is to consider that from results of invitro investigations cannot easily be concluded on invivo conditions. Influences on functional level, when even possible at all, can only hardly be simulated invitro [97]. Evidences grounding on invitro investigations can be entirely superposed by additional invivo regulations. As such, for example, expected effects by antioxidants could not be confirmed by whole animal investigation; by contrast, n-acetylcysteine even increased melanoma metastasis in mice [526]. However, this does not mean that knowledge of molecular coherences and induced signaling is of lower importance. Only must be recognized that a non-criticized invivo translation is not adequate.

Furthermore is to consider that cellular and molecular biologic studies describe only associations for the present. Questions on causality are open at first, but modifications of study construction can lead to coherences that make causality more probable. However, questions on adaptation and counter regulation often were left unanswered. Although cellular and molecular biologic intentions as well as the revealed signal pathways could be relevant for understanding the interconnections, one cannot really expect that such basic data are helpful in individual therapy monitoring and that can be used for therapy valuation overall. This is just in contrast to valuations by changes of autonomic function. So far, the two forms of investigations are not reciprocal excluding (if is disregarded that the provided means can be spent once only).

From the so observed outcome relevant alterations of autonomic function may surely result more far-reaching consequences. Accordingly to performing of studies should be questioned whether clinical investigations should not always be accompanied by Holter ECGs, and such already in phase 1 and phase 2. By this way could be differentiated, for example, whether an increase of sympathovagal balance can be referred to sympathetic activation or to vagal depression, possibly on the ground of diminished autonomic modulation in total [527]. Especially the last constitution was often connected with the increase of several severe diseases. And the knowledge of such condition can be got at early stage [528]. So it is not impossible that relative unsafe phase 3 studies with great patient size and finally unfavorable result overall can be reduced. However, this would further mean that ethic commitees must define the respectice control procedures. Likewise, clincans and statisticians must evaluate from what HRV change an adverse event is to conclude and from what a hospital admission is necessary for patients´ saftety.

HOWEVER, WHY HRV ANALYSIS DID NOT GET ADEQUATE ACCEPTANCE UNTIL NOW?

Upon the already published results that vagal activity was connected with good outcome and such measurement is not burdening for the patient, one should really surprise that the aspect of functional alteration is not adequately taken into pharmacological consideration, especially if the safety of drugs or the advantage in comparison to established drugs is concerned. First hints on pharmacological relevance are given in 1993 [200]. Currently, indeed cardiovascular risks by drugs are in the focus of the responsible lisence authorities. But cardiovascular complications are not the sole problems. Accordingly must be considered that impairment of central autonomic function may also lead to further diseases that are reducing the survival. As such, it can be thoroughly assumed that a lot of complications can be referred to typical autonomic alterations that can be ascertained non-invasively. And it must be required what can argue against such additional monitoring at all.

When thinking about, the question why alterations in autonomic response are only little recognized, surely should be multifarious. At first, every new investigation idea finds it hard to be accepted also because the diciding persons are typically beyond of middle age and have usually problems with fundamental news. For, if a serious new investigation field can be added, this is chargeable to the established ones. Next is to consider that rather higher costs must be awaited when more complicated patients can be better steered and therefore will longer survive. By the aim that costs shall be rather reduced one cannot really surprise that the engagement by the public side is rather restricted.

Also from the industy no impulses can be expected because a more extended monitoring during clinical studies would increase the costs, and although this is not required by the authorithies. Additionally must be reckoned that marketing of new agents can become aggravated, whereas the situation in older but licensed substances may be worse and a subsequent exploration is not prescribed. Further one cannot expect that the industry would push the research of unspecific influences. And conducting of such investigation independently from industry should not be clever as well, although this was already suggested [529, 530]. For, such studies would be interpreted as industry hostile and therefore the amount of industry sponsoring will decrease in that location.

Last but not least must be supposed from the side of physicians that such will not be promoted that serves for more transparency. For, the more you know, the more you can make wrong, and such creates points of attack. Similarly, networks in the form of an electronical health card, for example, were rather hampered by official physicians in Germany [531]. Therefore, surely the patient should be the only one who has interest in knowledge of his outcome relevant autonomic function. But the single concerned patient has no lobby and sometimes is already too weak for articulation. And the often mentioned problem of data safety can be avoided by self conducting or by patients´ individual dicision. Only when telemetric care will be conducted, data management should be performed with caution. However, in strictly consideration this aspect should be of minor relevance if severe ill patients are concerned. As such, the obsolute safety of data should not have priority by using this method e.g., for a 75 year old patient with diabetes mellitus and preterminal renal insufficiency. This patient tries only to live as long as possible.

Furthermore, such severe ill patients will get information by autonomic function measurement that may support the patient in participating of therapy dicision. Official this is wanted [532] although the daily work may become more complicated. However, this intention should get to more importance. Accordingly, e.g., in cancer diseases was pointed out that not only should be looked on relapse free intervals but also on severe complications that are reducing the survival [533]. Further should be clear that many oncologic agents are exerting different effects on antonomic function. From this fact can be concluded that by HRV monitoring, for example, less effective and rather dangerous therapy regimes should be objectively demasked. Therefore, unavantageous and superfluous treatment can be avoided by using this method.

Similar may hold true in the use of metformin in diabetics with renal insufficiency (s. above), because contraindication should be rather referred to pharmacokinetic problems [534] than to pharmacodynamic specialities. This could mean that dose reduction with differentiating monitoring may help to clarify whether the therapeutic benefit can perhaps overtop the risks (s. above) [211]. However, we cannot overlook the conflicting industry interests.

Nevertheless, not only physical insufficiencies can be estimated bei HRV but probably also the cognitive competence. According faculties were found to be associated with higher vagal activity, with faster reaction time, with more expressed stress intolerance as well as with greater oxygen consumption [106, 535, 536], and inversely with inflammatory reaction [537, 538]. So it is imaginable – and this must be extremely realized – that rather healthy and rather efficient collectives can be generated by measuring the individual autonomic nervous function. This surely can be interesting for employers and for life-insurances. However, church representatives and social associations should be more terrified at such potency.

Therefore, one must seriously reflect whether such possible examination is wanted by the society at all. However, the answer could consistently mean that an advantageous therapeutic monitoring would perhaps be restricted in severe ill patients. So, what is really more important? This must be anticipated and abundantly discussed – although, realistically, the dicision is not in question anymore. For, pandora´s box has been opened; a backward to yesterday is not imaginable. And what is possible should be done elsewhere, already when considering the modern pulse wristbands. Therefore, it should be more adequate when we are anticipating the facts and are taking part constructively. And when reflecting vagal activity, it is quite plausible that, for example, frequency of cancer as well as complications after the diagnosis of cancer may be reduced already by changing of lifestyle and nourishment in relevant extent [539].

LIMITATIONS AND SUPPLEMENTARY EXAMINATIONS

Impairing influences for themselves can be good explored when all other relevant co-factors are quite equal distributed. Recognition of significance, if is present, depends only on severity of effect and case number. However, much more interesting is the question how the single influences must be valued mutually. In other words, for example: What is more impairing the organism, alcohol use or air pollution? Which amount of daily alcohol intake is equivanlent to more or less constant air pollution? Similar should hold true for drugs. And on principle, measurement of autonomic alteration under defined provocation; e.g., HRV analysis at the tilt table, may reveal more detailed information.

However, whether consequences from the published rudimentary results can be formulated, is not clear until now. An imaginable progress in accordance to induction of special therapy today is only speculative. For getting more evidence, at first data on imaginable circumstances should be required by that advantages for the patient can be expected. Only after one had learned from this, the application of the method may be extended. For, alterations of autonomic function are quite unspecific at first. Furthermore should be awaited that changes in the therapeutic range should be rather low. Only in the sum of all influences (genetic determination [540], environment factors [541], nourishment [27], psychic burden [542] etc.) autonomic constellations may occur that would lead to a less centrally influenced situation in the individual patient. And this labil state can favor the development of diverse pathophysiological disarrangements that may end fatal more probably. Hence, valuation of autonomic and, especially, of vagal functions is very important under employment conditions too [543]. However, because is unknown what aim range should be aspired, the actual main question has not been answered until now.

Furthermore, one should not have only one method in view, because limitations and misinterpretations must be expected if valuation is entirely restricted to one instrument. For securing the relevance of findings the repertoire of non-invasive procedures should be extended to pulse wave velocity [544, 545], to heart rate recovery after defined provocation [546], to blood glucose variation (spontaneous vs. controlled) [547-552], to oxygen supply [553-556], to positron emission tomography [334, 557] and to a battery of other autonomic tests [558]. Beyond of, also combinations by the aid of EEG are very promising [559]. And examination and valuation of prolonged QTc interval has been already established [560, 561]. All these methods is common that they are reliably reflecting the autonomic modulation. A relevant interconnection of increased CRP, decreased HRV and QTc prolongation can be well assumed [562, 563].

However, HRV analysis may perhaps be preferred because vagal response can be estimated most specificly, as far as the patients are not too much arrhythmic or were supplied by a pace-maker. By this condition the autonomic state can be measured by usually available personnel computers by nearly everyone when instructions were given [2]. Arising costs are relative low and safety of data is ensured because results remain by the patient at first. Everybody himself decides on the extent of passing on.

CONCLUSION

Several facts are underlining the assumption that relevant unspecific effects may act on the autonomic and immunologic level. Hence, a reduced vagal function measured by HRV analysis or the herewith negatively associated anti-inflammation and NO delivery should be responsible for a lot of complications. Such are elevating the risk for premature death. Therefore, one must be aware that beyond autonomic function in general, especially vagal parts of autonomic nervous system should not be stressed unnecessarily. On the other side, the prognosis should be improved in several circumstances when vagal influences would have become intentionally elevated. In this concern it can be thoroughly assumed that the pharmacological potential should be promising, but surely more by the precondition that the respective aim corridor is known. Overall, therapy regimes should be valued on more than one aspect. In this the causal treatment may be improved by simultaneous optimizing the autonomic function.

Conflicts of Interest: None declared

REFERENCES

[1] Wang Shu-Ho. The Pulse Classic: Translation of the Maijing (ca. 220 A.D.), *Blue Poppy Press* 2000.

[2] Fleischer, J.; Nielsen, R.; Laugesen, E.; Nygaard, H.; Poulsen, PL. and Ejskjaer, N. (2011) Self-monitoring of cardiac autonomic function at home is feasible. *J. Diabetes Sci. Technol.* 5, 107-12.

[3] Sztajzel, J.; Jung, M. and Bayes de Luna, A. (2008) Reproducibility and gender-related difference of heart rate variability during all-day activity in young men and women. *Ann. Noninvasive Electrocardiol.* 13, 270-7.

[4] N.N. (1996) Heart rate variability: standards of measurement, physiological interpretation and clinical use. Task Force of the European Society of Cardiology and the North American Society of Pacing and Electrophysiology. *Circulation* 93, 1043-65.

[5] Elghozi, J.L.; Laude, D. and Girard, A. (1991). Effects of respiration on blood pressure and heart rate variability in humans. *Clin. Exp. Pharmacol. Physiol.* 18, 735–42.

[6] Julien, C. (2006) The enigma of Mayer waves: Facts and models. *Cardiovasc. Res.*, 70, 12–21.

[7] Sandercock, G.R. and Brodie, D.A. (2006) The role of heart rate variability in prognosis for different modes of death in chronic heart failure. *Pacing Clin Electrophysiol.* 29, 892-904.

[8] Pop-Busui, R.; Evans, G.W.; Gerstein, H.C.; Fonseca, V.; Fleg, J.L.; Hoogwerf, B.J.; Genuth, S.; Grimm, R.H.; Corson, M.A. and Prineas, R. (2010) Effects of cardiac autonomic dysfunction on mortality risk in the Action to Control Cardiovascular Risk in Diabetes (ACCORD) trial. *Diabetes Care* 33, 1578-84.

[9] Akselrod, S.; Gordon, D.; Ubel, F.A.; Shannon, D.C.; Berger, A.C. and Cohen, R.J. (1981) Power spectrum analysis of heart rate fluctuation: a quantitative probe of beat-to-beat cardiovascular control. *Science* 213, 220-2.

[10] Kleiger, R.E.; Miller, JP.; Bigger, J.T. Jr. and Moss, A.J. (1987) Decreased heart rate variability and ist association with increased mortality after acute myocardial infarction. *Am. J. Cardiol.* 59, 256-62.

[11] Malliani, A.; Lombardi, F.; Pagani, M. and Cerutti, S. (1994) Power spectral analysis of cardiovascular variability in patients at risk for sudden cardiac death. *J. Cardiovasc. Electrophysiol.* 5, 274-86.

[12] Stein, P.K.; Bosner, M.S.; Kleiger, R.E. and Conger, B.M. (1994) Heart rate variability: a measure of cardiac autonomic tone. *Am. Heart J.* 127, 1376-81.

[13] Villareal, R.P.; Liu, B.C. and Massumi, A. (2002) Heart rate variability and cardiovascular mortality. *Curr. Atheroscler. Rep.* 4, 120-7.

[14] Weise, F.; Krell, D. and Brinkhoff, N. (1986) Acute alcohol ingestion reduces heart rate variability. *Drug Alcohol. Depend.* 17, 89-9.

[15] Gonzalez Gonzalez, J.; Mendez Llorens, A.; Mendez Novoa, A. and Cordero Valeriano, J.J. (1992) Effect of acute alcohol ingestion on short-term heart rate fluctuations. *J. Stud. Alcohol.* 53, 86-90.

[16] Baumert, J.H.; Frey, A.W. and Adt, M. (1995) [Analysis of heart rate variability. Background, method, and possible use in anesthesia]. *Anaesthesist* 44, 677-86.

[17] Tsuji, H.; Venditti, F.J. Jr.; Manders, E.S.; Evans, J.C.; Larson, M.G.; Feldman, CL. and Levy, D. (1994) Reduced heart rate variability and mortality risk in an elderly cohort. The Framingham Heart Study. *Circulation* 90, 878-83.

[18] Dekker, J.M.; Schouten, E.G.; Klootwijk, P.; Pool, J.; Swenne, C.A. and Kromhout, D. (1997) Heart rate variability from short electrocardiographic recordings predicts mortality from all causes in middle-aged and elderly men. The Zutphen Study. *Am. J. Epidemiol.* 145, 899-908.

[19] Kröhnert, S. and Karsch, M. (2011) Sterblichkeit und Todesursachen. Online-Handbuch Demografie, Berlin-Institut für Bevölkerung und Entwicklung. http://www.berlin-institut.org/fileadmin/user_upload/handbuch_texte/pdf_Kroehnert_Karsch_Mortalitaet_2011.pdf.

[20] Wu, L.; Schaid, D.J.; Sicotte, H.; Wieben, E.D.; Li, H. and Petersen, G.M. (2015) Case-Only exome sequencing and complex disease susceptibility gene discovery: study design considerations, *J. Med. Genet.* 52, 10-6.

[21] Bredholt, G.; Mannelqvist, M.; Stansson, I.M.; Birkeland, E.; Hellem Bø, T.; Øyan, A.M.; Trovik, J.; Kalland, K.H.; Jonassen, I.; Salvesen, H.B.; Wik, E. and Akslen, L.A. (2015) Tumor necrosis is an important hallmark of aggressive endometrial cancer and associates with hypoxia, angiogenesis and inflammation responses. *Oncotarget* 6, 39676-91.

[22] Nolan, R.P.; Kamath, M.V.; Floras J.S.; Stanley, J.; Pang, C.; Picton, P. and Young, Q.R. (2005) Heart rate variability biofeedback as a

behavioral neurocardiac intervention to enhance vagal heart rate control. *Am. Heart J.* 149, 1137.

[23] Hamer, M. and Steptoe, A. (2007) Association between physical fitness, parasympathetic control, and proinflammatory responses to mental stress. *Psychosom Med.* 69, 660-6.

[24] Luttmann-Gibson H1, Suh HH, Coull BA, Dockery DW, Sarnat SE, Schwartz J, Stone PH, Gold DR (2010) Systemic inflammation, heart rate variability and air pollution in a cohort of senior adults. *Occup. Environ. Med.* 67, 625-30.

[25] Li, X.; Feng, Y.; Deng, H.; Zhang, W.; Kuang, D.; Deng, Q.; Dai, X.; Lin, D.; Huang, S.; Xin, L.; He, Y.; Huang, K.; He, M.; Guo, H.; Zhang, X. and Wu, T. (2012) The dose-response decrease in heart rate variability: any association with the metabolites of polycyclic aromatic hydrocarbons in coke oven workers? *PLoS One* 7, e44562.

[26] Hansen, A.L.; Dahl, L.; Olson, G.; Thornton, D.; Graff, I.E.; Frøyland, L.; Thayer, J.F. and Pallesen, S. (2014) Fish consumption, sleep, daily functioning, and heart rate variability. *J. Clin. Sleep Med.* 10, 567-75.

[27] Park, S.K.; Tucker, K.L.; O'Neill, M.S.; Sparrow, D.; Vokonas, P.S.; Hu, H. and Schwartz, J. (2009) Fruit, vegetable, and fish consumption and heart rate variability: the Veterans Administration Normative Aging Study. *Am. J. Clin. Nutr.* 89, 778-86.

[28] Souza, B.B.; Monteze, N.M.; de Oliveira, F.L.; de Oliveira, J.M.; de Freitas Nascimento, S.; Marques do Nascimento Neto, R.; Sales. M.L. and Souza, G.G. (2014) Lifetime shift work exposure: association with anthropometry, body composition, blood pressure, glucose and heart rate variability. *Occup. Environ. Med.* 72, 208-15.

[29] Huang, J.; Deng, F.; Wu, S.; Lu, H. and Guo, X. (2013) The effects of short-term exposure to noise and traffic-related air pollution on heart rate variability in young healthy adults. *J. Expo. Sci. Environ. Epidemiol.* 23, 559-564.

[30] Kraus, U.; Schneider, A.; Breitner, S.; Hampel, R.; Rückerl, R.; Pitz, M.; Geruschkat, U.; Belcredi, P.; Radon, K. and Peters, A. (2013) Individual daytime noise exposure during routine activities and heart rate variability in adults: a repeated measures study. E*nviron. Health Perspect.* 121, 607-12.

[31]   Wallin, B.G. (2007) Interindividual differences in muscle sympathetic nerve activity: a key to new insight into cardiovascular regulation? *Acta Physiol. (Oxf.)* 190, 265-75.

[32]   Asanoi, H. (2009) [Application of microneurography to circulatory disorders]. *Brain Nerve* 61, 270-6.

[33]   Wulsin, L.R.; Horn, P.S.; Perry, J.L.; Massaro, J.M. and D'Agostino, R.B. (2015) Autonomic Imbalance as a Predictor of Metabolic Risks, Cardiovascular Disease, Diabetes, and Mortality. J. *Clin. Endocrinol. Metab.* 100, 2443-8.

[34]   Saito. I.; Hitsumoto, S.; Maruyama, K.; Nishida, W.; Eguchi, E.; Kato, T.; Kawamura, R.; Takata, Y.; Onuma, H.; Osawa, H. and Tanigawa, T. (2015) Heart rate variability, insulin resistance, and insulin sensitivity in Japanese adults: The Toon Health Study. *J. Epidemiol.* 25, 583-91.

[35]   Kardelen, F.; Akçurin, G.; Ertuğ, H.; Akcurin, S. and Bircan, I. (2006) Heart rate variability and circadian variations in type 1 diabetes mellitus. *Pediatr. Diabetes* 7, 45-50.

[36]   Lehnen, A.M.; Leguisamo, N.M.; Casali, K.R. and Schaan, B.D. (2013) Progressive cardiovascular autonomic dysfunction in rats with evolving metabolic syndrome. *Auton. Neurosci.* 176, 64-9.

[37]   Süfke, S.; Djonlagić, H. and Kibbel, T. (2010) [Impairment of cardiac autonomic nervous system and incidence of arrhythmias in severe hyperglycemia]. *Med. Klin. (Munich)* 105, 858-70.

[38]   Stockhorst, U.; Huenig, A.; Ziegler, D. and Scherbaum, W.A. (2011) Unconditioned and conditioned effects of intravenous insulin and glucose on heart rate variability in healthy men. *Physiol. Behav.* 103, 31-8.

[39]   Sayk, F.; Vietheer, A.; Schaaf, B.; Wellhoener, P.; Weitz, G.; Lehnert, H. and Dodt, C. (2008) Endotoxemia causes central downregulation of sympathetic vasomotor tone in healthy humans. *Am. J. Physiol. Regul. Integr. Comp. Physiol.* 295, R891-8.

[40]   Saito, I.; Hitsumoto, S.; Maruyama, K.; Eguchi, E.; Kato, T.; Okamoto, A.; Kawamura, R.; Takata, Y.; Nishida, W.; Nishimiya, T.; Onuma, H.; Osawa, H. and Tanigawa, T. (2015) Impact of heart rate variability on C-reactive protein concentrations in Japanese adult nonsmokers: The Toon Health Study. *Atherosclerosis* 244, 79-85.

[41]   Cooper, T.M.; McKinley, P.S.; Seeman, T.E.; Choo, T.H.; Lee, S. and Sloan, R.P. (2015) Heart rate variability predicts levels of inflammatory

markers: Evidence for the vagal anti-inflammatory pathway. *Brain Behav. Immun.* 49, 94-100.

[42] Chen, W.L. and Kuo, C.D. (2007) Characteristics of heart rate variability can predict impending septic shock in emergency department patients with sepsis. *Acad. Emerg. Med.* 14, 392-7.

[43] Pontet, J.; Contreras, P.; Curbelo, A.; Medina, J.; Noveri, S.; Bentancourt, S. and Migliaro, E.R. (2003) Heart rate variability as early marker of multiple organ dysfunction syndrome in septic patients. *J. Crit. Care* 18, 156-63.

[44] Korach, M.; Sharshar, T.; Jarrin, I.; Fouillot, J. P.; Raphaël, J. C.; Gajdos, P., and Annane, D. (2001) Cardiac variability in critically ill adults: Influence of sepsis. *Crit. Care Med.* 29, 1380-1385.

[45] Barnaby, D.; Ferrick, K.; Kaplan, D. T.; Shah, S.; Bijur, P., and Gallagher, E. J. (2002) Heart rate variability in emergency department patients with sepsis. *Acad. Emerg. Med.* 9, 661-670.

[46] Jaiswal, M.; Urbina, E.M.; Wadwa, R.P.; Talton, J.W.; D´Agostino, R.B. Jr.; Hamman, R.F.; Fingerlin, T.E.; Daniels, S.; Marcovina, S.M.; Dolan, L.M. and Dabelea, D. (2013) Reduced heart rate variability among youth with type 1 diabetes: the SEARCH CVD study. *Diabetes Care* 36, 157-62.

[47] Turker, Y.; Aslantas, Y.; Aydin, Y.; Demirin, H.; Kutlucan, A.; Tibilli, H.; Turker, Y. and Ozhan, H. (2013) Heart rate variability and heart rate recovery in patients with type 1 diabetes mellitus. *Acta Cardiol.* 68, 145-50.

[48] Pal, G.K.; Adithan, C.; Ananthanarayanan, P.H.; Pal, P.; Nanda, N.; Durgadevi, T.; Lalitha, V.; Syamsunder, A.N. and Dutta, T.K. (2013) Sympathovagal imbalance contributes to prehypertension status and cardiovascular risks attributed by insulin resistance, inflammation, dyslipidemia and oxidative stress in first degree relatives of type 2 diabetics. *PLoS One* 8, e78072.

[49] Tarvainen, M.P.; Lipponen, J.A.; Al-Aubaidy, H. and Jelinek, H.F. (2012) Effect of hyperglycemia on cardiac autonomic function in type 2 diabetes. *Comput. Cardiol.* 39, 405-408.

[50] Chyun, D.A.; Wackers, F.J.; Inzucchi, S.E.; Jose, P.; Weiss, C.; Davey J.A.; Heller, G.V.; Iskandrian, A.E. and Young, L.H. (2015). Autonomic dysfunction independently predicts poor cardiovascular outcomes in

asymptomatic individuals with type 2 diabetes in the DIAD study. *SAGE Open Medicine*, 2015 Feb 24.

[51] Feng, Y.; Sun, H.; Song, Y.; Bao, J.; Huang, X.; Ye, J.; Yuan, J.; Chen, W.; Christiani, D.C.; Wu, T. and Zhang, X. (2014) A community study of the effect of polycyclic aromatic hydrocarbon metabolizes on heart rate variability based on the Framingham risk score. *Occup. Environ. Med.* 71, 338-45.

[52] Süfke, S.; Djonlagic´, H. and Kibbel, T. (2008) [Continuous analysis of heart rate variability for examination of cardiac autonomic nervous system after doxepin intoxication]. *Intensivmed.* 45 121–31.

[53] Süfke, S.; Fiedler, S.; Djonlagiç, H. and Kibbel, T. (2009) [Continuous analysis of heart rate variability for examination of cardiac autonomic nervous system after alcohol intoxication]. *Med. Klin. (Munich)* 104, 511-9.

[54] Bau, P.F.; Moraes, R.S.; Bau, C.H.; Ferlin, E.L.; Rosito, G.A. and Fuchs, F.D. (2011) Acute ingestion of alcohol and cardiac autonomic modulation in healthy volunteers. *Alcohol* 45, 123-9.

[55] Nessler, J.; Nessler, B.; Kitliński, M.; Libionka. A.; Kubinyi, A.; Konduracka, E. and Piwowarska, W. (2007) Sudden cardiac death risk factors in patients with heart failure treated with carvedilol. *Kardiol. Pol.* 65, 1417-22.

[56] Ozdemir, M.; Arslan, U.; Türkoğlu, S.; Balcioğlu, S. and Cengel, A. (2007) Losartan improves heart rate variability and heart rate turbulence in heart failure due to ischemic cardiomyopathy. *J. Card. Fail.* 13, 812-7.

[57] Tanindi, A.; Olgun, H.; Celik, B. and Boyaci, B. (2012) Heart rate variability in patients hospitalized for decompensated diastolic heart failure at admission and after clinical stabilization. *Future Cardiol.* 8, 473-82.

[58] Huang, J.L.; Wen, Z.C.; Lee, W.L.; Chang, M.S. and Chen, S.A. (1998) Changes of autonomic tone before the onset of paroxysmal atrial fibrillation. *Int. J. Cardiol.* 66, 275-83.

[59] Fioranelli, M.; Piccoli, M.; Mileto, G.M.; Sgreccia, F.; Azzolini, P.; Risa, M.P.; Francardelli, R.L.; Venturini, E. and Puglisi, A. (1999) Analysis of heart rate variability five minutes before the onset of paroxysmal atrial fibrillation. *Pacing Clin. Electrophysiol.* 22, 743-9.

[60] Lombardi, F.; Tarricone, D.; Tundo, F.; Colombo, F.; Belletti, S. and Fiorentini, C. (2004) Autonomic nervous system and paroxysmal atrial fibrillation: a study based on the analysis of RR interval changes before, during and after paroxysmal atrial fibrillation. *Eur. Heart J.* 25, 1242-8.

[61] Tomita, T.; Takei, M.; Saikawa, Y.; Hanaoka, T.; Uchikawa, S.; Tsutsui, H.; Aruga, M.; Miyashita, T.; Yazaki, Y.; Imamura, H.; Kinoshita, O.; Owa, M. and Kubo, K. (2003) Role of autonomic tone in the initiation and termination of paroxysmal atrial fibrillation in patients without structural heart disease. *J. Cardiovasc. Electrophysiol.* 14, 559-64.

[62] Markos, F.; Snow, H.M.; Kidd, C. and Conlon, K. (2001) Inhibition of neuronal nitric oxide reduces heart rate variability in the anaesthetised dog. *Exp. Physiol.* 86, 539-41.

[63] Choate, J.K.; Danson, E.J.; Morris, J.F. and Paterson, D.J. (2001) Peripheral vagal control of heart rate is impaired in neuronal NOS knockout mice. *Am. J. Physiol. Heart Circ. Physiol.* 281, H2310-7.

[64] Kalla, M.; Chotalia, M.; Hao, G. and Herring, N. (2015) Acetylcholine analogue mimics the protective effect of cardiac vagal nerve stimulation on ventricular fibrillation threshold. *Eur Heart J.* 34 (Suppl. 1), P5021.

[65] Han, X.; Kobzik, L.; Zhao, Y.Y.; Opel, D.J.; Liu, W.D.; Kelly, R.A. and Smith, T.W. (1997) Nitric oxide regulation of atrioventricular node excitability. *Can. J. Cardiol.* 13, 1191-201.

[66] Musialek, P.; Lei, M.; Brown, H.F.; Paterson, D.J. and Casadei, B. (1997) Nitric oxide can increase heart rate by stimulating the hyperpolarization-activated inward current, I(f). *Circ. Res.* 81, 60-8.

[67] Bosch, T.A.; Kaufman, C.L.; Williamson, E.B.; Duprez, D.A. and Dengel, D.R. (2009) Comparison of changes in heart rate variability and blood pressure during nitroglycerin administration and head-up tilt testing. *Clin. Auton. Res.* 19, 46-50.

[68] Kibbel, T. (2007) Akute Veränderungen des neurovegetativen Tonus´ bei intravenöser Molsidomin- oder Nitroglycerin-Applikation - Randomisierte doppelblinde Crossover-Studie mittels Herzfrequenz variabilitäts-Analyse und Plasma-Katecholaminbestimmung. Thesis, Universität zu Lübeck, http://www.zhb.uni-luebeck.de/epubs/ediss267.pdf.

[69] Tracey, K.J. (2002) The inflammatory reflex. *Nature* 420, 853-9.

[70] Lu, H.L.; Ouyang, W. and Huang, C. (2006) Inflammation, a key event in cancer development. *Mol. Cancer Res.* 4, 221-33.

[71]   Rakoff-Nahoum, S. (2006) Why cancer and inflammation? *Yale J. Biol. Med.* 79, 123-30.

[72]   Colotta, F.; Allavena, P.; Sica, A.; Garlanda, C. and Mantovani, A. (2009) Cancer-related inflammation, the seventh hallmark of cancer: links to genetic instability. *Carcinogenesis* 30, 1073-81.

[73]   Grivennikov, S.I.; Greten, F.R. and Karin, M. (2010) Immunity, inflammation, and cancer. *Cell* 140, 883-99.

[74]   Adams, S.C.; Schondorf, R.; Benoit, J. and Kligour. R.D. (2015) Impact of cancer and chemotherapy on autonomic nervous system function and cardiovascular reactivity in young adults with cancer: a case-controlled feasibility study. *B.M.C. Cancer* 15, 414.

[75]   Cancer Research UK, Cancer Incidence by Age (2015) http://www.cancerresearchuk.org/health-professional/cancer-statistics/incidence/age.

[76]   Umetani, K.; Singer, D.H.; McCraty, R. and Atkinson, M. (1998) Twenty-four hour time domain heart rate variability and heart rate: relations to age and gender over nine decades. *J. Am. Coll. Cardiol.* 31, 593-601.

[77]   Kuo, T.B.; Lin, T.; Yang, C.C.; Li, C.L.; Chen, C.F. and Chou, P. (1999) Effect of aging on gender differences in neural control of heart rate. *Am. J. Physiol.* 277, H2233-9.

[78]   Sun, P.; Zhou, K.; Wang, S.; Li, P.; Chen, S.; Lin, G.; Zhou, Y. and Wang, T. (2013) Involvement of MAPK/NF-κB signaling in the activation of the cholinergic anti-inflammatory pathway in experimental colitis by chronic vagus nerve stimulation. *PLoS One* 8, e69424.

[79]   Chen, C.F.; Lai, C.L.; Lin, H.F.; Liou, L.M. and Lin, R.T. (2011) Reappraisal of heart rate variability in acute ischemic stroke. *Kaohsiung J. Med. Sci.* 27, 215-21.

[80]   Xiong, L.; Leung, H.W.; Chen, X.Y.; Leung, W.H.; Soo, O.Y. and Wong, K.S. (2014) Autonomic dysfunction in different subtypes of post-acute ischemic stroke. *J. Neurol. Sci.* 337, 141-6.

[81]   Zhang, Y.; Popovic, Z.B.; Bibevski, S.; Fakhry, I.; Sica, D.A.; Van Wagoner, D.R. and Mazgalev, T.N. (2009) Chronic vagus nerve stimulation improves autonomic control and attenuates systemic inflammation and heart failure progression in a canine high-rate pacing model. *Circ. Heart Fail.* 2, 692-9.

[82] De Ferrari, G.M. and Schwartz, P.J. (2011) Vagus nerve stimulation: from pre-clinical to clinical application: challenges and future directions. *Heart Fail. Rev.* 16, 195-203.

[83] Li, W. and Olshansky, B. (2011) Inflammatory cytokines and nitric oxide in heart failure and potential mudulation by vagus nerve stimulation. *Heart Fail. Rev.* 16, 137-45.

[84] Cooper, T.M.; McKinley, P.S.; Seeman, T.E.; Choo, T.; Lee, S. and Sloan, R.P. (2014) Heart rate variability predicts levels of inflammatory markers: Evidence for vagal anti-inflammatory pathway. B*rain Behav. Immun.* 49, 94-100.

[85] Shacter, E. and Weitzman, S. (2002) Chronic inflammation and cancer. *Oncology (Williston Park)* 16, 217-26, 229.

[86] Coussens, L.M. and Werb, Z. (2002) Inflammation and cancer. *Nature* 420, 860-7.

[87] Newton, J.L.; Allen, J.; Kerr, S. and Jones, D.E. (2006) Reduced heart rate variability and baroreflex sensitivity in primary biliary cirrhosis. *Liver Int.* 26, 197-202.

[88] Ghia, J.E.; Blennerhassett, P.; Kumar-Ondiveeran, H.; Verdu, E.F. and Collins, S.M. (2006) The vagus nerve: a tonic inhibitory influence associated with inflammatory bowel disease in a murine model. *Gastroenterology* 131, 1122-30.

[89] Goldstein, R.S.; Bruchfeld, A.; Yang, L.; Qureshi, A.R.; Gallowitsch-Puerta, M.; Patel, N.B.; Huston, B.J.; Chavan, S.; Rosas-Ballina, M.; Gregersen, P.K.; Czura, C.J.; Sloan, R.P.; Sama A.E. and Tracey, K.J. (2007) Cholinergic anti-inflammatory pathway activity and High Mobility Group Box-1 (HMGB1) serum levels in patients with rheumatoid arthritis. *Mol. Med.* 13, 210-5.

[90] Harnod, D.; Wen, S.H.; Chen, S.Y. and Harnod, T. (2014) The association of heart rate variability with parkinsonian motor symptom duration. *Yonsei Med. J.* 55, 1297-302.

[91] Ferini-Strambi, L.; Rovaris, M.; Oldani, A.; Martinelli, V.; Filippi, M.; Smirne, S.; Zucconi, M. and Comi, G. (1995) Cardiac autonomic function during sleep and wakefulness in multiple sclerosis. *J. Neurol.* 242, 639-43.

[92] Allan, L.M., Ballard, C.G.; Allen, J.; Murray, A.; Davidson, A.W. McKeith, I.G. and Kenny, R.A. (2007) Autonomic dysfunction in dementia. *J. Neurol. Neurosurg. Psychiatry* 78, 671-7.

[93]   Sarkis, R.A.; Thome-Souza, S.; Poh, M.Z.; Llewellyn, N.; Klehm. J.; Madsen, J.R.; Picard, R.; Pennell, P.B.; Dworetzky, B.A.; Loddenkemper, T. and Reinsberger, C. (2015) Autonomic changes following generalized tonic clonic seizures: An analysis of adult and pediatric patients with epilepsy. *Epilepsy Res.* 115, 113-8.

[94]   Chen, C.F.; Lin, H.F.; Lin, R.T.; Yang, Y.H. and Lai, C.L. (2013) Relationship between ischemic stroke location and autonomic cardiac function. *J. Clin. Neurosci.* 20, 406-9.

[95]   Birkhofer, A.; Schmidt, G. and Förstl, H. (2005) [Heart and brain – the influence of psychiatric disorders and their therapy on the heart rate variability]. *Fortschr. Neurol. Psychiatr.* 73, 192-205.

[96]   Boettger, S.; Hoyer, D.; Falkenhahn, K.; Kaatz, M.; Yeragani, V.K. and Bär, K.J. (2006) Altered diurnal autonomic variation and reduced vagal information flow in acute schizophrenia. *Clin. Neurophysiol.* 117, 2715-22.

[97]   Galow, L.V.; Schneider, J.; Lewen, A.; Ta, T.T.; Papageorgiou, I.E., and Kann, O. (2014) Energy substrates that fuel fast neuronal network oscillations. *Front. Neurosci.* 8, 398.

[98]   Pavlov, V.A. and Tracey, K.J. (2005) The cholinergic anti-inflammatory pathway. *Brain Behav. Immun.* 19, 493-9.

[99]   Das, U.N. (2011) Vagus nerve stimulation as a strategy to prevent and manage metabolic syndrome. *Med. Hypotheses* 76, 429-33.

[100] Meregnani, J.; Clarençon, D.; Vivier, M.; Peinnequin, A.; Mouret, C.; Sinniger, V.; Picq, C.; Job, A.; Canini, F.; Jacquier-Sarlin, M. and Bonaz, B. (2011) Anti-inflammatory effect of vagus nerve stimulation in a rat model of inflammatory bowel disease. *Auton. Neurosci.* 160, 82-9.

[101] Abboud, F.M.; Harwani, S.C. and Chapleau, M.W. (2012) Autonomic neural regulation oft he immune system: Implications for hypertension and cardiovascular disease. *Hypertension* 59, 755-62.

[102] Bertolini, A. (2012) Drug-induced activation of the nervous control of inflammation: a novel possibility for the treatment of hypoxic damage. *Eur. J. Pharmacol.* 679, 1-8.

[103] Houston, J.M. (2012) The vagus nerve and the inflammatory reflex: wandering on a new treatment paradigm for systemic inflammation and sepsis. *Surg. Infect. (Larchmt.),* 13, 187-93.

[104] Boeckxstaens, G. (2013) The clinical importance of the anti-inflammatory vagovagal reflex. *Handb. Clin. Neurol.* 117, 119-34.

[105] Gaspari, R.J. and Paydarfar, D. (2014) Pulmonary effects of intravenous atropine induce ventilation perfusion mismatch. *Can. J. Physiol. Pharmacol.* 92, 399-404.

[106] Hansen, A.L.; Johnsen, B.H. and Thayer, J.F. (2003) Vagal influence on working memory and attention. *Int. J. Psychophysiol.* 48, 263-74.

[107] Perna, L.; Wahl, H.W.; Mons, U.; Saum, K.U.; Holleczek, B. and Brenner, H. (2015) Cognitive impairment, all-cause and cause-specific mortality among non-demented older adults. *Age Ageing* 44, 445-51.

[108] Psychari, S.N.; Apostolou, T.S.; Iliodromitis, E.K.; Kourakos, P.; Liakos, G. and Kremastinos, D.T. (2007) Inverse relation of C-reactive protein levels to heart rate variability in patients after acute myocardial infarction. *Hellenic J. Cardiol.* 48, 64-71.

[109] Haarala, A.; Kähönen, M.; Eklund, C.; Jylhävä, J.; Koskinen, T.; Taittonen, L.; Huupponen, R.; Lehtimäki, T; Viikari, J.; Raitakari, O.T. and Hurme, M. (2011) Heart rate variability is independently associated with C-reactive protein but not with Serum amyloid A. The Cardiovascular Risk in Young Finns Study. Eur. *J. Clin. Invest.* 41, 951-7.

[110] Jarczok, M.N.; Koenig, J.; Mauss, D.; Fischer, J.E. and Thayer, J.F. (2014) Lower heart rate variability predicts increased level of C-reactive protein 4 years later in healthy, nonsmoking adults. *J. Intern. Med.* 276, 667-71.

[111] De Couck, M.; Mravec, B. and Gidron, Y. (2012) You may need the vagus nerve to understand pathophsiology and to treat diseases. *Clin. Sci. (Lond.)* 122, 323-8.

[112] Mouten, C.; Ronson, A.; Razavi, D.; Delhaye, F.; Kupper, N.; Paesmans, M.; Moreau, M.; Nogaret, J.M.; Hendlisz, A. and Gidron, Y. (2012) The relationship between heart rate variability and time-course of carcinoembryonic antigen in colorectal cancer. *Auton. Neurosci.*, 166, 96-9.

[113] Gidron, Y.; De Couck, M. and De Greve, J. (2014) If you have an active vagus nerve, cancer stage may no longer be important. *J. Biol. Regul. Homeost. Agents* 28, 195-201.

[114] Giese-Davis, J.; Wilhelm, F.H.; Tamagawa, R.; Palesh, O.; Neri, E.; Taylor, C.B.; Kraemer, H.C. and Spiegel, D. (2015) Higher vagal activity as related to survival in patients with advanced breastcancer: an analysis of autonomic dysregulation. *Psychosom.* 77, 346-55.

[115] Ebbehøj, E.; Poulsen, P.L.; Hansen, K.W.; Knudsen, S.T.; Mølgaard, H. and Mogensen, C.E. (2002) Effects on heart rate variability of metoprolol supplementary to ongoing ACE-inhibitor treatment in type I diabetic patients with abnormal albuminuria. *Diabetologia* 45, 965-75.

[116] Rajab, M.; Jin, H.; Welzig, C.M.; Albano, A.; Aronovitz, M.; Zhang, Y.; Park, H.J.; Link, M.S.; Noujaim, S.F. and Galper, J.B. (2013) Increased inducibility of ventricular tachycardia and decreased heart rate variability in a mouse model for type 1 diabetes: effect of pravastatin. *Am. J. Physiol. Heart Circ. Physiol.* 305, H1807-16.

[117] Al-Khaled, M.; Matthis, C. and Eggers, J. (2014) Statin treatment in patients with acute ischemic stroke. *Int. J. Stroke* 9, 597-601.

[118] Kin, J.; Kwak, H.J.; Cha, J.Y.; Jeong, Y.S.; Rhee, S.D.; Kim. K.R. and Cheon, H.G. (2014) Metformin suppresses lipopolysaccharide (LPS)-induced inflammatory response in murine macrophages via activating transcription factor-3 (ATF-3) induction. *J. Biol. Chem.* 289, 13246-55.

[119] Othman, A.A.; Abou Rayia, D.M.; Ashour, D.S.; Saied, E.M.; Zineldeen, D.H. and El-Ebiary, A.A. (2015) Atorvastatin and metformin administration modulates experimental Trichinella spiralis infection. *Parasitol. Int.* 65, 105-112.

[120] Ou, S.Y.; Chu, H.; Chao, P.W.; Ou, S.M.; Lee, Y.J.; Kuo, S.C.; Li, S.Y.; Shih, C.J. and Chen, Y.T. (2014) Effect of the use of low and high potency statins and sepsis outcomes. *Intensive Care Med.* 40, 1509-17.

[121] Ahern, T.P.; Pedersen, L.; Tarp, M.; Cronin-Fenton, D.P.; Garne, J.P.; Silliman, R.A.; Sørensen, H.T. and Lash, T.L. (2011) Statin prescriptions and breast cancer recurrence risk: a Danish nationwide prospective cohort study. *J. Natl. Cancer Inst.* 103, 1461-8.

[122] Baur, D.M.; Klotsche, J.; Hamnvik, O.P.; Sievers, C.; Pieper, L.; Wittchen, H.U.; Stalla, G.K.; Schmid, R.M.; Kales, S.N. and Mantzoros, C.S. (2011) Type 2 diabetes mellitus and medications for type 2 diabetes mellitus are associated with risk for and mortality from cancer in a German primary care cohort. *Metabolism* 60, 1363-71.

[123] Holmes, M.D. and Chen, W.Y. (2012) Hiding in plain view: the potential for commonly used drugs to reduce breast cancer mortality. *Breast Cancer Res.* 14, 216.

[124] Franciosi, M.; Lucisano, G.; Lapice, E.; Strippoli, C.F.; Pellegrini, F. and Nicolucci, A. (2013) Metformin therapy and risk of cancer in patients with type 2 diabetes: systematic review. *PLoS One* 8, e71583.

[125] Pimentel, M.A.; Chai, M.G.; Le, C.P.; Cole, S.W. and Sloan, E.K. (2013) Sympathetic nervous system regulation of metastasis. *Madame Curie Bioscience Database, Landes Bioscience,* http://www.ncbi.nlm.nih.gov/books/NBK5974/.

[126] Li, W.; Wang, Q.L.; Liu, X.; Dong, S.H.; Li, H.X.; Li, C.Y.; Guo, L.S.; Gao, J.M.; Berger, N.A.; Li, L.; Ma, L. and Wu, Y.J. (2015) Combined use of vitamin D3 and metformin exhibits synergistic chemopreventive effects on colorectal neoplasia in rats and mice. *Cancer Prev. Res. (Phila.)* 8, 139-48.

[127] Zhong, S.; Zhang, X.; Chen, L.; Ma, T.; Tang, J. and Zhao, J. (2015) Statin use and mortality in cancer patients: Systematic review and meta-analysis of observational studies. *Cancer Treat. Rev.* 41, 554-67.

[128] Zhong, S.; Yu, D.; Zhang, X.; Chen, X.; Yang, S.; Tang, J.; Zhao, J. and Wang, S. (2015) ß-Blocker use and mortality in cancer patients: systematic review and meta-analysis of observational studies. *Eur. J. Cancer Prev.*, 2015 Sep 3.

[129] Chen, C.I.; Kuan, C.F.; Fang, Y.A.; Liu, S.H.; Liu, J.C.; Wu, L.L.; Chang, C.J.; Yang, H.C.; Hwang, J.; Miser, J.S. and Wu, S.Y. (2015) Cancer risk in HBV patients with statin and metformin use: a population-based cohort study. *Medicine (Baltimore)* 94, e462.

[130] Svensson, M., Schmidt, E.B.; Jørgensen, K.A. and Christensen, J.H. (2007) The effect of n-3 fatty acids on heart rate variability in patients treated with chronic hemodialysis. *J. Ren. Nutr.* 17, 243-9.

[131] Christensen, J.H. (2011) Omega-3 polyunsaturated fatty acids and heart rate variability. *Front. Physiol.* 2, 84.

[132] Valera, B.; Suhas, E.; Counil, E.; Poirier, P. and Dewailly, E. (2014) Influence of polyunsaturated fatty acids on blood pressure, resting heart rate and heart rate variability among French Polynesians. *J. Am. Coll. Nutr.* 33, 288-96.

[133] Akita, M.; Kuwahara, M.; Itoh, F.; Nakano, Y.; Osakabe, N.; Kurosawa, T. and Tsubone, H. (2008) Effects of cacao liquor polyphenols on cardiovascular and autonomic nervous functions in hypercholsterolaemic rabbits. *Basic Clin. Pharmacol. Toxicol.* 103, 581-7.

[134] Rodríguez-Ramiro, I.; Ramos, S.; López-Oliva, E.; Agis-Torres, A.; Bravo, L.; Goya, L. and Martin, M.A. (2013) Cocao polyphenols prevent inflammation in the colon of azoxymethane-treated rats and in TNF-α-stimulated Caco-2-cells. *Br. J. Nutr.* 110, 206-15.

[135] Aires, V.; Limagne, E.; Cotte, A.K.; Latruffe, N.; Ghiringhelli, F. and Delmas, D. (2013) Resvaltrol metabolites inhibit human metastatic colon cancer cells progression and synergize with chemotherapeutic drugs to induce cell death. *Mol. Nutr. Food Res.* 57, 1170-81.

[136] Ivey, K.L.; Hodgson, J.M.; Croft, K.D.; Lewis, J.R. and Prince, R.L. (2015) Flavonoid intake and all-cause mortality. *Am. J. Clin. Nutr.* 101, 1012-20.

[137] Lai, C.S.; Wu, J.C.; Ho, C.T. and Pan, M.H. (2015) Disease chemopreventive effects and molecular mechanisms of hydroxylated polymethoxyflavones. *Biofactors* 41, 301-13.

[138] Ulgen, M.S.; Akdemir, O. and Toprak, N. (2001) The effects of trimetazidine on heart rate variability and signal-averaged electrocardiography in early period of acute myocardial infarction. *Int. J. Cardiol.* 77, 255-62.

[139] Topal, E.; Ozdemir, R.; Barutcu; I.; Aksoy, Y.; Sincer, I.; Akturk, E. and Cehreli, S. (2006) The effects of trimetazidine on heart rate variability in patients with slow coronary artery flow. *J. Electrocardiol.* 39, 211-8.

[140] Gunes, Y.; Guntekin, U.; Tuncer, M. and Sahin, M. (2009) The effects of trimetazidine on heart rate variability in patients with heart failure. *Arq. Bras. Cardiol.* 93, 154-8.

[141] Tallarico, D.; Rizzo, V.; DiMaio, F.; Petretto, F.; Bianco, G.; Placanica, G.; Marziali, V.; Gueli, N.; Meloni, F. and Campbell, S.V. (2003) Myocardial cytoprotection by trimetazidine against anthracycline-induced toxicity in anticancer chemotherapy. *Angiology* 54, 219-27.

[142] Salouege, I.; Ben Ali, R.; Ben Saïd, D.; Elkadri, N.; Kourda, N.; Lakhal, M. and Klouz, A. (2014) Means of evaluation and protection from doxorubicin-induced cardiotoxicity and hepatotoxicity in rats. *J. Cancer Res. Ther.* 10, 274-8.

[143] De Meersman, R.E.; Zion, A.S.; Lieberman, J.S. and Downey, J.A. (2000) Acetylsalicylic acid and autonomic modulation. *Clin. Auton. Res.* 10, 197-201.

[144] Durmaz, T.; Keles, T.; Ozdemir, O.; Bayram, N.A.; Akcay, M.; Yeter, E. and Bozkurt, E. (2008) Heart rate variability in patients with stable coronary artery disease and aspirin resistance. *Int. Heart J.* 49, 413-22.

[145] Majumdar, A.P.; Banerjee, S.; Nautiyal, J.; Patel, B.B.; Patel, V.; Du, J.; Yu, Y.; Elliott, A.A.; Levi, E. and Sarkar, F.H. (2009) Curcumin

synergizes with resveratrol to inhibit colon cancer. *Nutr. Cancer* 61, 544-53.

[146] Pongchaidecha, A.; Lailerd, N.; Boonprasert, W. and Chattipakorn, N. (2009) Effects of curcuminoid supplement on cardiac autonomic status in high-fat-induced obese rats. *Nutrition* 25, 870-8.

[147] Thangapazham, R.L.; Passi, N. and Maheshwari, R.K. (2007) Green tea polyphenol and epigallocatechin gallate induce apoptosis and inhibit invasion in human breast cancer cells. *Cancer Biol. Ther.* 6, 1938-43.

[148] Huang, Y.Q.; Lu, X.; Min, H.; Wu, Q.Q.; Shin, X.T.; Bian, K.Q. and Zou, X.P. (2016) Green tea and liver cancer risk: A meta-analysis of prospective cohort studies in Asian populations. *Nutrition* 32, 3-8.

[149] Renehan, A.G.; Roberts, D.L. and Dive, C. (2008) Obesity and cancer: pathophysiological and biological mechanisms. *Arch. Physiol. Biochem.* 114, 71-83.

[150] De Pergola, G. and Silvestris, F. (2013) Obesity as a major risk factor for cancer. *J. Obes.* 2013, 291546.

[151] Sánchez, R.C., Ibáñez, C. and Klaassen, J. (2014) [The link between obestity and cancer]. *Rev. Med. Chil.* 142, 211-21.

[152] Indumathy, J.; Pal, G.K.; Pal, P.; Ananthanarayanan, P.H.; Parija, S.C.; Balachander, J. and Dutta, T.K. (2015) Association of sympathovagal imbalance with obesity indices, and abnormal metabolic biomarkers and cardiovascular parameters. *Obes. Res. Clin. Pract.* 9, 55-6.

[153] Ziegler, D.; Strom, A.; Nowotny. B.; Zahiragic, L.; Nowotny, P.J.; Carstensen-Kirberg, M.; Herder, C. and Roden, M. (2015) Effect of low-energy diets differing on fiber, red meat, and coffee intake on cardiac autonomic function in obese individuals with type 2 diabetes. *Diabetes Care* 38, 1750-7.

[154] Daniłowicz-Szymanowicz, L.; Figura-Chmielewska, M.; Ratkowski, W. and Raczak, G. (2013) Effect of various forms of physical training on the autonomic nervous system activity in patients with acute myocardial infarction. *Kardiol. Pol.* 71, 558-65.

[155] Galetta, F.; Franzoni, F.; Tocchini, L.; Camici, M.; Milanesi, D.; Belatti, F.; Speziale, G.; Rossi, M.; Gaudio, C.; Carpi, A. and Santoro, G. (2013) Effect of physical activity on heart rate variability and carotid intima-media thickness in older people. *Intern. Emerg. Med.* 8 (Suppl 1), S27-9.

[156] Kang, D.; Kim, Y.; Kim, J.; Hwang, Y.; Cho, B.; Hong, T.; Sung, B. and Lee, Y. (2015) Effects of high occupational physical activity, aging, and

exercise on heart rate variability among male workers. *Ann. Occup. Environ. Med.* 27, 22.

[157] Zhang, T.; Guo, P.; Zhang, Y.; Xiong, H.; Yu, X.; Wang, X.; He, D. and Jin, X. (2013) The antidiabetic drug metformin inhibits the proliferartion of bladder cells in vitro and in vivo. *Int. J. Mol. Sci.* 14, 24603-18.

[158] Nangia-Makker, P.; Yu, Y.; Vasudevan, A.; Farhana, L.; Rajendra, S.G.; Levi, E. and Majumdar, A.P. (2014) Metformin: a potential therapeutic agent for recurrent colon cancer. *PLoS One* 9, e84369.

[159] Bergheim, I.; Luyendyk, J.P.; Steele, C.; Russell, G.K.; Guo. L.; Roth, R.A. and Arteel, G.E. (2006) Metformin prevents endotoxin-induced liver injury after partial hepatectomy. *J. Pharmacol. Exp. Ther.* 316, 1053-61.

[160] Bhat, A.; Sebastiani, G. and Bjat, M. (2015) Systematic review: Preventive and therapeutic applications of metformin in liver disease. *World J. Hepatol.* 7, 1652-9.

[161] Koh, S.J.; Kim, J.M.; Kim, I.K.; Ko, S.H. and Kim, J.S. (2014) Anti-inflammatory mechanism of metformin and its effects in intestinal inflammation and colitis-associated colon cancer. *J. Gastroenterol. Hepatol.* 29, 502-10.

[162] Kang, K.Y.; Kim, Y.K.; Yi, H.; Kim, J.; Jung, H.R.; Kim, I.J.; Cho, J.H.; Park, S.H.; Kim, H.Y. and Ju, J.H. (2013) Metformin downregulates Th17 cells differentiation and attenuates murine autoimmune arthritis. *Int. Immunopharmacol.* 16, 85-92.

[163] Son, H.J.; Lee, J.; Lee, S.Y.; Kim, E.K.; Park, M.J.; Kim, K.W.; Park, S.H. and Cho, M.L. (2014) Metformin attenuates experimental autoimmune arthritis through reciprocal regulation of Th17/Treg balance and osteoclastogenesis. *Mediators Inflamm.* 2014, 973986.

[164] Yan, H.; Zhou, H.F.; Hu, Y. and Pham, C.T. (2015) Suppression of experimental arthritis through AMP-activated protein kinase activation and autophagy modulation. *J. Rheum. Dis. Treat.* 1, 5.

[165] Wahlqvist, M.L.; Lee, M.S.; Hsu, C.C.; Chuang, S.Y.; Lee, J.T. and Tsai, H.N. (2012) Metformin-inclusive sulfonylurea therapy reduces the risk of Parkinson´s disease occurring with type 2 diabetes in a Taiwanese population cohort. *Parkinsonism Relat. Disord.* 18, 753-8.

[166] Patil, S.P.; Jain, P.D.; Ghumatkar, P.J.; Tambe, R. and Sathaye, S. (2014) Neuroprotective effect of metformin in MPTP-induced Parkinson´s disease in mice. *Neuroscience* 277, 747-54.

[167] Nath, N.; Khan, M.; Paintlia, M.K.; Singh, I.; Hoda, M.N. and Giri, S. (2009) Metformin attenuated the autoimmune disease of the central nervous system in animal models of multiple sclerosis. *J. Immunol.* 182, 8005-14.

[168] Paintlia, A.S.; Mohan, S. and Singh, I. (2013) Combinatorial effect of metformin and lovastatin impedes T-cell autoimmunity and neurodegeneration in experimental autoimmune encephalomyelitis. *J. Clin. Cell. Immunol.* 4, 10.4172/2155-9899.1000149.

[169] Zhao, R.R.; Xu, X.C.; Xu, F.; Zhang, W.L.; Liu, L.M. and Wang, W.P. (2014) Metformin protects against seizures, learning and memory impairments and oxidative damage induced by pentylenetetrazole-induced kindling in mice. *Biochem. Biophys. Res. Commun.* 448, 414-7.

[170] Chen, C.F.; Lin, H.F.; Lin, R.T.; Yang, Y.H. and Lai, C.L. (2013) Relationship between ischemic stroke location and autonomic cardiac function. *J. Clin. Neurosci.* 20, 406-9.

[171] Jin, Q.; Cheng, J.; Liu, Y.; Wu, J.; Wang, X.; Wei, S.; Zhou, X.; Qin, Z.; Jia, J. and Zhen, X. (2014) Improvement of functional recovery by chronic metformin treatment is associated with enhanced alternative of microglia/macrophages and increased angiogenesis and neurogenesis following experimental stroke. *Brain Behav. Immun.* 40, 131-42.

[172] Li. J.; Benashshki, S.E.; Venna, V. and McCullough, L.D. (2010) Effects of metformin in experimental stroke. *Stroke* 41, 2645-52.

[173] Protti, A.; Fortunato, F.; Monti, M.; Vecchio, S.; Gatti, S.; Comi, G.P.; De Giuseppe, R. and Gattinoni, L. (2012) Metformin overdose, but not lactic acidosis per se, inhibits oxygen consumption in pigs. *Crit. Care* 16, R75.

[174] Lin, H.C.; Stein, J.D.; Nan, B.; Childers, G.; Newman-Casey, P.A.; Thompson, D.A. and Richards, J.E. (2015) Association of geroprotective effects of metformin and risk of open-angle dlaucoma in patients with diabetes mellitus. *JAMA Opthalmol.* 133, 915-23.

[175] Glutz, A.; Leitmeyer, K.; Setz, C.; Brand, Y. and Bodmer, D. (2015) Metformin protects auditory hair cells from gentamicin-induced toxicity in vitro. *Audiol. Neurootol.* 20, 360-9.

[176] Ng, E.H.; Wat, N.M. and Ho, P.C. (2001) Effects of metformin on ovulation rate, hormonal and metabolic profiles in women with clomiphene-resistant polycystic ovaries: a randomized, double-blinded placebo-controlled trial. *Hum. Reprod.* 16, 1625-31.

[177] Makled, A.K.; El Sherbiny, M. and Elkabarity, R. (2014) Assessment of ovarian stromal blood flow after metformin treatment in women with polycystic ovary syndrome. *Arch. Gynecol. Obstet.* 289, 883-91.

[178] Hsu, C.C.; Wahlqvist, M.L.; Lee, M.S. and Tsai, H.N. (2011) Incidence of dementia is increased in type 2 diabetes and reduced by the use of sulfonylureas and metformin. *J. Alzheimers Dis.* 24, 485-93.

[179] Ng, T.P.; Feng, L.; Yap, K.B.; Lee, T.S.; Tan, C.H. and Winblad, B. (2014) Long-term metformin usage and cognitive function among older adults with diabetes. *J. Alzheimers Dis.* 41, 61-8.

[180] Moore, E.M.; Mander, A.G.; Ames, D.; Kotowicz, M.A.; Carne, R.P.; Brodaty, H.; Woodward, M.; Boundy, K.; Ellis, K.A.; Bush, A.I.; Faux, N.G.; Martins, R.; Szoeke, C.; Rowe. C. and Watters, D.A. (2013) Increased risk of cognitive impairment in patients with diabetes is associated with metformin. *Diabetes Care* 36, 2981-7.

[181] Goodarzi, M.O. (2014) Comment on Moore et al. Increased risk of cognitive impairment in patients with diabetes is associated with metformin. Diabetes Care 2013. *Diabetes Care* 37, e150.

[182] Chen, Y.; Zhou, K.; Wang, R.; Liu, Y.; Kwak, YD.; Ma, T.; Thompson, R.C.; Zhao, Y.; Smith, L.; Gasparini, L.; Luo, Z.; Xu, H, and Liao, F.F. (2009) Antidiabetic drug metformin (Glucophage®) increases biogenesis of Alzheimer´s amyloid peptides via up-regulating BACE1. *Proc. Natl. Acad. Sci. USA.* 106, 3907-12.

[183] DiTacchio, K.A.; Heinemann, S.F. and Dziewczapolski, G. (2015) Metformin treatment alters memory function in a mouse model of Alzheimer´s disease. *J. Alzheimers Dis.* 44, 43-8.

[184] Bonnefont-Rousselot, D.; Raji, B.; Walrand, S.; Gardès-Albert, M.; Jore, D.; Legrand, A.; Peynet, J. and Vasson, M.P. (2003) An intracellular modulation of free radical production could contribute to the beneficial effects of metformin towards oxidative stress. *Metabolism* 52, 586-9.

[185] Wu, C.L.; Qiang, L.; Han, W.; Ming, M.; Viollet, B. and He, Y.Y. (2013) Role of AMPK in UVB-induced DNA damage repair and growth control. *Oncogene* 32, 2682-9.

[186] Lehraiki, A.; Abbe, P.; Cerezo, M.; Rounaud, F.; Regazzetti, C.; Chignon-Sicard, B.; Passeron, T.; Bertolotto, C.; Ballotti, R. and Rocchi, S. (2014) Inhibition of melanogenesis by the antidiabetic metformin. *J. Invest. Dermatol.* 134, 2589-97.

[187] Shaw, R.J. (2006) Glucose metabolism and cancer. *Curr. Opin. Cell. Biol.* 18, 598-608.

[188] Garcia-Heredia, J.M.; Felipe-Abrio, B.; Cano, D.A. and Carnero, A. (2015) Genetic modification of hypoxia signaling in animal models and its effect on cancer. *Clin. Transl. Oncol.* 17, 90-102.

[189] Chen, S.; Zhu, X.; Lai. X.; Xiao, T.; Wen, A. and Zhang, J. (2014) Combined cancer therapy with non-conventional drugs: all roads lead to AMPK. *Mini Rev. Med. Chem.* 14, 642-54.

[190] Zhao, M.; Sun, L.; Yu, X.J.; Miao, Y.; Liu, J, J.; Wang, H.; Ren, J. and Zang, W.J. (2013) Acetylcholine mediates AMPK-dependent autophagic cytoprotection in H9c2 cells during hypoxia/reoxygenation injury. *Cell. Physiol. Biochem.* 32, 601-13.

[191] Martinez-Outschoorn, U.; Sotgia, F. and Lisanti, M.P. (2014) Tumor microenvironment and metabolic synergy in breast cancers: critical importance of mitochondrial fuels and function. *Semin. Oncol.* 41, 195-216.

[192] Hirsch, H.A.; Iliopoulos, D. and Struhl, K. (2013) Metformin inhibits the inflammatory response associated with cellular transformation and cancer stem cell growth. *Proc. Natl. Acad. Sci. USA* 110, 972-7.

[193] Hettich, M.M.; Matthes, F.; Ryan, D.P.; Griesche, N.; Schröder, S.; Dorn, S.; Krauß, S. and Ehninger, D. (2014) The anti-diabetic drug metformin reduces BACE1 protein level by interfering with the MID1 complex. *PLoS One* 9, e102420.

[194] Kim, M.H.; Kim, M.O.; Heo, J.S.; Kim, J.S. and Han, H.J. (2008) Acetylcholine inhibits long-term hypoxia-induced apoptosis by suppressing the oxidative stress-mediated MAPKs activation as well as regulation of Bcl-2, c-IAPs, and caspase-3 in mouse embryonic stem cells. *Apoptosis* 13, 295-304.

[195] Miao, Y.; Zhou, J.; Zhao, M.; Liu, J.; Sun, L.; Yu, X.; He, X.; Pan, X. and Zang, W. (2013) Acetylcholine attenuates hypoxia/reoxygenation-induced mitochondrial and cytosolic ROS formation in H9c2 cells via M2 acetylcholine receptor. *Cell. Physiol. Biochem.* 31, 189-98.

[196] Matteoli, G.; Gomez-Pinilla, P.J.; Nemethova, A.; Di Giovangiulio, M.; Cailotto, C.; van Bree. S.H.; Michel, K.; Tracey, K.J.; Schemann, M.; Boesmans, W.; Vanden Berghe, P. and Boeckxstaens, G.E. (2014) A distinct vagal anti-inflammatory pathway modulates intestinal

muscularis resident macrophages independent of the spleen. *Gut* 63, 938-48.

[197] Bao, B.; Ahmad, A.; Kong, D.; Ali, S.; Azmi, A.S.; Li, Y.; Banerjee, S.; Padhye, S. and Sarkar, F.H. (2012) Hypoxia induced aggressiveness of prostate cancer cells is linked with deregulated expression of VEGF, IL-6 and miRNAs that are attenuated by CDF. *PLoS One* 7, e43726.

[198] Jia, J.; Cheng, J.; Ni, J. and Zhen, X. (2015) Neuropharmacological actions of metformin in stroke. *Curr. Neuropharmacol.* 13, 389-94.

[199] Manzella, D.; Grella, R.; Esposito, K.; Giugliano, D.; Barbagallo, M. and Paolisso, G. (2004) Blood pressure and cardiac autonomic nervous system in obese type 2 diabetic patients: effect of metformin administration. *Am. J. Hypertens.* 17, 223-7.

[200] van Ravenswaaij-Arts, C.M.; Kollée, L.A.; Hopman, J.C.; Stoelinga, G.B. and van Geijn, H.P. (1993) Heart rate variability. *Ann. Intern. Med.* 118, 436-47.

[201] Routledge, H.C.; Chowdhary, S. and Townend, J.N. (2002) Heart rate variability--a therapeutic target? *J. Clin. Pharm. Ther.* 27, 85-92.

[202] Chen, X.; Walther, F.J.; Sengers, R.M.; Laghmani, el H.; Salam, A.; Folkerts, G.; Pera, T. and Wagenaar, G.T. (2015) Metformin attenuates hyperoxia-induced lung injury in neonatal rats by reducing the inflammatory response. *Am. J. Physiol. Lung. Cell. Mol. Physiol.* 309, L262-70.

[203] Learsi, S.K.; Bastos-Silva, V.J.; Lima-Silva, A.E.; Bertuzzi, R. and De Araujo, G.G. (2015) Metformin improves performance in high-intensity exercise, but not anaerobic capacity in healthy male subjects. *Clin. Exp. Pharmacol. Physiol.* 42, 1025-9.

[204] Williams, E.D.; Rogers, S.C.; Zhang, X.; Azhar, G. and Wei, J.Y. (2015) Elevated oxygen consumption rate in response to acute low-glucose stress: Metformin restores rate to normal level. *Exp. Gerontol.* 70, 157-62.

[205] Glenn, T.C.; Kelly, D.F.; Boscardin, W.J.; McArthur, D.L.; Vespa, P.; Oertel, M.; Hovda, D.A.; Bergsneider, M.; Hillered, L. and Martin, N.A. (2003) Energy dysfunction as a predictor of outcome after moderate or severe head injury: indices of oxygen, glucose, and lactate metabolism. *J. Cereb. Blood Flow Metab.* 23, 1239-50.

[206] Kin, J.; Kwak, H.J.; Cha, J.Y.; Jeong, Y.S.; Rhee, S.D.; Kim, K.R. and Cheon, H.G. (2014) Metformin suppresses lipopolysaccharide (LPS)-

induced inflammatory response in murine macrophages via activating transcription factor-3 (ATF-3) induction. *J. Biol. Chem.* 289, 13246-55.

[207] Singhal, A.; Jie, L.; Kumar, P.; Hong, G.S.; Leow, M.K.; Paleja, B.; Tsenova, L.; Kurepina, N.; Chen, J.; Zolezzi, F.; Kreiswirth, B.; Poidinger, M.; Chee, C.; Kaplan, G.; Wang, Y.T. and De Libero, G. (2014) Metformin as adjunct antituberculosis therapy. Sci. Transl. Med. 6, 263ra159.

[208] Hung, S.C.; Chang, Y.K.; Liu, J.S.; Kuo, K.L.; Chen, Y.H.; Hsu, C.C. and Tarng, D.C. (2015) Metformin use and mortality in patients with advanced chronic kidney disease: national, retrospective, observational, cohort study. *Lancet Diabetes Endocrinol.* 3, 605-14.

[209] Deligiannis, A.; Kouidi, E. and Tourkantonis, A (1999) Effects of physical training on heart rate variability in patients on hemodialysis. *Am. J. Cardiol.* 84, 197-202.

[210] Galetta, F.; Cupisti, A.; Franzoni, F.; Morelli, E.; Caprioli, R.; Rindi, P. and Barsotti, G. (2001) Changes in heart rate variability in chronic uremic patients during ultrafiltration and hemodialysis. *Blood Purif.* 19, 395-400.

[211] Heaf, J. (2014) Metformin in chronic kidney disease: time for a rethink. *Perit. Dial. Int.* 34, 353-7.

[212] Orban, J.C.; Fontaine, E. and Ichai, C. (2012) Metformin overdose: time to move on. *Crit. Care* 16, 164.

[213] Grau, I.; Ardanuy, C.; Calatayud, L.; Schulze, M.H.; Liñares, J and Pallares R (2014) Smoking and alcohol abuse are the most preventable risk factors for invasive pneumonia and other pneumococcal infections. *Int. J. Infect. Dis.* 25, 59-64.

[214] Bala, S.; Marcos, M.; Gattu, A.; Catalano, D. and Szabo, G. (2014) Acute binge drinking increases serum endotoxin and bacterial DNA levels in healthy individuals. *PLoS One* 9, e96864.

[215] Cogliano, V.J.; Baan, R.; Straif, K.; Grosse, Y.; Lauby-Secretan, B.; El Ghissassi, F.; Bouvard, V.; Benbrahim-Tallaa, L.; Guha, N.; Freeman, C.; Galichet, L.; Wild, C.P. (2011) Preventable exposures associated with human cancers. *J. Natl. Cancer Inst.* 103, 1827-39.

[216] Bagnardi, V.; Blangiardo, M.; La Vecchia, C. and Corrao, G. (2001) Alcohol Consumption and risk of cancer: a meta-analysis. *Alcohol Res. Health* 25, 263-70.

[217] Homann, N.; Stickel, F.; König, I.R.; Jacobs. A.; Junghanns, K.; Benesova, M.; Schuppan, D.; Himsel, S.; Zuber-Jerger, I.; Hellerbrand, C.; Ludwig, D.; Caselmann, W.H. and Seitz, H.K. (2006) Alcohol dehydrogenase 1C*1 allele is a genetic marker for alcohol-associated cancer in heavy drinkers. *Int. J. Cancer* 118, 1998-2002.

[218] Diamond, B.J., Kim, H.; DeLuca, J. and Cordero, D.L. (1995) Cardiovascular regulation in multiple sclerosis. *Mult. Scler.* 1, 156-62.

[219] Monge-Argilés, J.A.; Palacios-Ortega, F.; Vila-Sobrino, J.A. and Matias-Guiu, J. (1998) Heart rate variability in multiple sclerosis during a stable phase. *Acta Neurol. Scand.* 97, 86-92.

[220] Devos, D.; Kroumova, M.; Bordet, R.; Vodougnon, H.; Gulieu, J.D.; Libersa, C. and Destee, A. (2003) Heart rate variability and Parkinson´s disease severity. *J. Neural. Transm.* 110, 997-1011.

[221] Lotufo, P.A.; Valliengo, L.; Benseñor, I.M. and Brunoni, A.R. (2012) A systematic review and meta.analysis of heart rate variability in epilepsy and antiepileptic drugs. *Epilepsia*, 53, 272-82.

[222] Ponnusamy, A.; Marques, J.L. and Reuber, M. (2012) Comparison of heart rate variability parameters during complex partial seizures and psychogenic nonepileptic seizures. *Epilepsia* 53 1314-21.

[223] Soares-Miranda, L.; Sattelmair, J.; Chaves, P.; Duncan, G.E.; Siscovick, D.S.; Stein, P.K. and Mozaffarian, D. (2014) Physical activity and heart rate variability in older adults. The Cardiovascular Health Study. *Circulation* 129, 2100-10.

[224] Süfke, S.; Djonlagic´, H. and Kibbel, T. (2015) Severe Sepsis and Septic Shock: Different Concepts of Analgesia and Sedation May Have Important Influences on Prognosis and Therapy Management. In: Benedict Graver (ed.) Septic Shock: Risk Factors, Management and Prognosis, Chapter 2, 27-60, Nova Science Publishers, Inc. New York.

[225] Siegmund-Schultze (2015) Nosokomialinfektionen mit multiresistenten Keimen – Acitenobacter auf dem Vormarsch. *Dtsch. Ärztebl.* 112, A184.

[226] Tallgren, M.; Pettilä, V. and Hynninen, M. (2006) Quality assessment of sedation in intensive care. *Acta Anaesthesiol. Scand.* 50, 942-6.

[227] Xing, X.Z.; Gao, Y.; Wang, H.J.; Qu, S.N.; Huang, C.L.; Zhang, H.; Wang, H.; Xiao, Q.L. and Sun, K.L. (2015) Effect of sedation on short-term and long-term outcomes of critically ill patients with acute respiratory insufficiency. *World J. Emerg. Med.* 6, 147-52.

[228] Minhas, M.A.; Velasquez, A.G.; Kaul, A.; Salinas, P.D. and Celi, L.A. (2015) Effect of Protocolized Sedation on Clinical Outcomes in Mechanically Ventilated Intensive Care Unit Patients: A Systematic Review and Meta-analysis of Randomized Controlled Trials. *Mayo Clin. Proc.* 90, 613-23.

[229] Burry, L.; Rose, L.; McCullagh, I.J.; Fergusson, D.A.; Ferguson, N.D. and Mehta, S. (2014) Daily sedation interruption versus no daily sedation interruption for critically ill adult patients requiring invasive mechanical ventilation. *Cochrane Database Syst. Rev.* 7, CD009176.

[230] Dwyer, D.J.; Belenky, P.A.; Yang, J.H.; MacDonald, I.C.; Martell, J.D.; Takahashi, N.; Chan, C.T.; Lobritz, M.A.; Braff, D.; Schwarz, E.G-; Ye, J.D.; Pati, M.; Vercruysse, M.; Ralifo, P.S.; Allison, K.R.; Khalil, A.S.; Ting, A.Y.; Walker, G.C. and Collins, J.J. (2014) Antibiotics induce redox-related physiological alterations as a part of their lethality. *Proc. Natl. Acad. Sci. USA* 111, E2100-E2109.

[231] Abdel-Salam, O.M.; Abdel-Rahman, R.F.; Sleem, A.A.; Mosry, F.A. and Sharaf, H. A. (2013) Effects of afferent and efferent denervation of vagal nerve on endotoxin-induced oxidative stress in rats. *J. Neural. Transm. (Vienna)* 120, 1673-88.

[232] Chen, M.; Zhou, X.; Yu, L.; Liu, Q.; Sheng, X.; Wang, Z.; Wang, S.; Jiang, H. and Zhou, S. (2015) Low-level vagus nerve stimulation attenuates myocardial ischemic reperfusion injury by antioxidative stress and antiapoptosis reactions in canines. *J. Cardiovasc. Electrophysiol.*, 2015 Oct 7.

[233] Chiarugi, M.; Buccianti, P.; Disarli, M.; Galatioto, C. and Cavina, E. (2000) Effect of blood transfusions on disease-free interval after rectal cancer surgery. *Hepatogastroenterology* 47, 1002-5.

[234] ARD-Mediathek (2014) "Böses Blut" – Transfusionsrisiken, Kehrtwende in der Intensivmedizin. http://www.ardmediathek.de/tv/odysso-Wissen-im-SWR/B%C3%B6ses-Blut-Gef%C3%A4hrliche-Bluttransfusion/SWR-Fernsehen/Video?documentId=26699558&bcas tId=246888, 2014 Nov 24.

[235] Jagoditsch, M.; Pozgainer, P.; Klingler, A. and Tschmelitsch, J. (2006) Impact of blood transfusions on recurrence and survival after rectal cancer surgery. *Dis. Colon Rectum* 49, 1116-30.

[236] Faber, J.C. and Hardin, S.R. (2010) Outcomes of knee replacement patients using autotransfusion. *Orthop. Nurs.* 29, 333-7.

[237] Koonrungsesomboon, N.; Tantiworawit, A.; Phrommintikul, A.; Saekho, S.; Srichairattanakool, S. and Chattipakorn, N. (2015) Heart rate variability for early detection of iron overload cardiomyopathy in ß-thalassemia patients. *Hemoglobin* 39, 281-6.

[238] Wijarnpreecha, K.; Siri-Angkul, N.; Shinlapawittayatorn, K.; Charoenkwan, P.; Silvilairat, S.; Siwasomboon, C.; Visarutratna, P.; Srichairatanakool. S.; Tantiworawit, A.; Phrommintikul, A; Chattipakorn, S.C. and Chattipakorn, N. (2015) Heart rate variability as an alternative indicator for identifying cardiac iron status in non-transfusion dependent thalassemia patients. *PLoS One* 10, e0130837.

[239] Thephinlap, C.; Phisalaphong, C.; Lailard, N.; Chattipakorn, M.; Winichagoon, P.; Vadolas, J.; Fucharoen, S.; Porter, J.B. and Srichairatanakool, S. (2011) Reversal of cardiac iron loading and dysfunction in thalassemic mice by curcuminoids. *Med. Chem.* 7, 62-9.

[240] Muller, L.M.; Gorter, K.J.; Hak, E.; Goudzwaard, W.L.; Schellevis, F.G.; Hoepelman, A.I. and Rutten, G.E. (2005) Increased risk of common infections in patients with type 1 and type 2 diabetes mellitus. *Clin. Infect. Dis.* 41, 281-8.

[241] Cleveland, R.J.; North, K.E.; Stevens, J.; Teitelbaum, S.L.; Neugut, A.I. and Gammon, M.D. (2012) The association of diabetes with breast cancer incidence and mortality in the Long Island Breast Cancer Study Project. *Cancer Causes Control* 23, 1193-203.

[242] Xu, H.L.; Fang, H.; Xu, W.H.; Qin, G.Y.; Yan, Y.J.; Yao, B.D.; Zhao, N.Q.; Liu, Y.N.; Zhang, F.; Li, W.X.; Wang, N.; Zhou, J.; Zhang, J.L.; Zhao, L.Y.; Li, L.Q. and Zhao, Y.P. Cancer incidence in patients with type 2 diabetes mellitus: a population-based cohort study in Shanghai. *B.M.C. Cancer* 15, 852.

[243] Wu, L.; Zhu, J.; Prokop, L.J. and Murad, M.H. (2015) Pharmacologic therapy of diabetes and overall cancer risk and mortality: A meta-analysis of 265 Studies. *Sci. Rep.* 5, 10147.

[244] Chiu, W.Y.; Shih, S.R. and Tseng, C.H. (2012) A review on the association between glucagon-like peptide-1 receptor agonists and thyroid cancer. *Exp. Diabetes Res.* 2012, 924168.

[245] Vasilakou, D.; Karagiannis, T.; Athanasiadou, E.; Mainou, M.; Liakos, A.; Bekiari, E.; Sarigianni, M.; Metthews, D.R. and Tsapas, A. (2013) Sodium.glucose cotransporter 2 inhibitors for type 2 diabetes: a systematic review and meta-analysis. *Ann. Intern. Med.* 159, 262-74.

[246] Nauck, M.A. (2014) Update on developments with SGLT2 inhibitors in the management of type 2 diabetes. *Drug Des. Devel. Ther.* 8, 1335-80.

[247] Lin, H.W. and Tseng, C.H. (2014) A review on the relationship between SGLT2 inhibitors and cancer. *Int. J. Endocrinol.* 2014, 719578.

[248] Nauck, M.A. and Friedrich, N. (2013) Do GLP-1-based therapies increase cancer risk? *Diabetes Care* 36 (Suppl. 2), S245-52.

[249] Berkelaar, M.; Eekhoff, E.M.; Simonis-Bik, A.M.; Boomsma, D.I.; Diamant, M.; Ijzerman, R.G.; Dekker, J.M.; 'tHart, L.M. and de Geus, E.J. (2013) Effects of induced hyperinsulinaemia with and without hyperglycemia on measures of cardiac vagal control. *Diabetologia* 56, 1436-43.

[250] Cherney, D.Z.; Perkins, B.A.; Soleymanlou, N.; Har, R.; Fagan, N.; Johansen, O.E., Woerle, H.J.; von Eynatten, M. and Broedl, U.C. (2014) The effect of empagliflozin on arterial stiffness and heart rate variability in subjects with uncomplicated type 1 diabetes mellitus. *Cardiovasc. Diabetol.* 13, 28.

[251] Griffioen, K.J.; Wan, R.; Okun, E.; Wang, X.; Lovett-Barr, M.R.; Li, Y.; Mughal, M.R.; Mendelowitz, D. and Mattson, M.P. (2011) GLP-1 receptor stimulation depresses heart rate variability and inhibits neurotransmission to cardiac vagal neurons. *Cardiovasc. Res.* 89: 72-8.

[252] Cherney, D.Z.; Perkins, B.A.; Soleymanlou, N.; Maione, M.M.; Lai, V.; Lee, A.; Fagan, N.M.; Woerle, H.J.; Johansen, O.E.; Broedl, U.C. and von Eynatten, M. (2014) Renal hemodynamic effect of sodium-glucose cotransporter 2 inhibition in patients with type 1 diabetes mellitus. *Circulation* 129, 587-97.

[253] Vasilakou, D.; Karagiannis, T.; Athanasiadou, E.; Mainou, M.; Liakos, A.; Bekiari, E.; Sarigianni, M.; Metthews, D.R. and Tsapas, A. (2013) Sodium glucose cotransporter 2 inhibitors for type 2 diabetes: a systematic review and meta-analysis. *Ann. Intern. Med.* 159, 262-74.

[254] Weir, M.R.; Januszewicz, A.; Gilbert, R.E.; Vijapurkar, U.; Kline, I.; Fung, A. and Meininger, G. (2014) Effect of canagliflocin on blood pressure and adverse events related to osmotic diuresis and reduced intravascular volume in patients with type 2 diabetes mellitus. *J. Clin. Hypertens.* 16, 875-82.

[255] Umegaki, H. and Khookhor, O. (2013) The response of the autonomic nervous system to the cholinestrase inhibitor, donepezil. *Neuro. Endocrinol. Lett.* 34, 383-7.

[256] Wolk, R.; Kulakowski, P. and Ceremuzynski, L. (1996) Nifedipine and captopril exert divergent effects on heart rate variability in patients with acute episodes of hypertension. *J. Hum. Hypertens.* 10, 327-332.

[257] Yamamoto, H.; Lee, C.E.; Marcus, J.N.; Williams, T.D.; Overton, J.M.; Lopez, M.E.; Hollenberg, A.N.; Baggio, L.; Saper, C.B.; Drucker, D.J. and Elmquist, J.K. (2002) Glucagon-like peptide-1 receptor stimulation increases blood pressure and heart rate and activates autonomic regulatory neurons. *J. Clin. Invest.* 110, 43-52.

[258] Valensi, P.; Chiheb, S. und Fysekidis, M. (2013) Insulin- and glucagon-like peptide-1-induced changes in heart rate and vagosympathetic activity: why they matter. *Diabetologia* 56, 1196-200.

[259] Schirra, J.; Houck, P.; Wank, U.; Arnold, R.; Göke, B. and Katschinski, M. (2000) Effects of glucagon-like peptide-1 (7-36) amide on antro-pyloro-duodenal lipid perfusion in humans. *Gut* 46, 622-31.

[260] Pannacciulli, N.; Bunt, J.C.; Koska, J.; Bogardus, C and Krakoff, J. (2006) Higher fasting plasma concentrations of glucagon-like peptide 1 are associated with higher resting energy expenditure and fat oxidation rates in humans. *Am. J. Clin. Nutr.* 84, 556-60.

[261] Lu, Z.; Percie Du Sert, N.; Chan, S.W.; Yeung, C.K.; Lin, G.; Yew, D.T.; Andrews, P.L. and Rudd, J.A. (2014) Differential hypoglycemic, anorectic, autonomic and emetic effects on the glucagon-like peptide receptor agonist, exendin-4, in the conscious telemetered ferret. *J. Trans. Med.* 12, 327.

[262] Valensi, P.; Chiheb, S. and Fysekidis, M. (2013) Insulin- and glucagon-like peptide-1-induced changes in heart rate and vagosympathetic activity: why they matter. *Diabetologia* 56, 1196-200.

[263] Apaijai, N.; Pintana, H.; Chattipakorn, S.C. and Chattipakorn, N. (2012) Cardioprotective effects of metformin and vildaglyptin in adult rats with insulin resistance induced by high-fat diet. *Endocrinology* 153, 3878-3885.

[264] Paolisso, G.; Manzella, D.; Tagliamonte, M.R.; Rizzo, M.R.; Gambardella, A. and Varricchio, M. (1999) Effects of different insulin infusion rates on heart rate variability in lean and obese subjects. *Metabolism* 48, 755-62.

[265] Bergholm, R.; Westerbacka, J.; Vehkavaara, S.; Seppälä-Lindroos, A.; Goto, T. and Yki-Järvinen, H. (2001) Insulin sensitivity regulates

autonomic control of heart rate variation independent of body weight in normal subjects. *J. Clin. Endocrinol. Metab.* 86, 1403-9.

[266] Galinier, M.; Fourcade, J.; Ley, N.; Boveda, S.; Solera, S.; Solera, M.L.; Massabuau, P.; Elhabaj, S.; Fauvel, J.M.; Valdiguié, P. and Bounhoure, J.P. (1999) [Hyperinsulinism, heart rate variability and circadian variation of arterial pressure in obese hypertensive patients]. *Arch. Mal. Coeur. Vaiiss.* 92, 1105-9.

[267] Stockhorst, U.; Huenig, A.; Ziegler, D. and Scherbaum, W.A. (2011) Unconditioned and conditioned effects of intravenous insulin and glucose on heart rate variability in healthy men. *Physiol. Behav.* 103, 31-8.

[268] Apaijai, N.; Pintana, H.; Chattipakorn, S.C. and Chattipakorn, N. (2012) Cardioprotective effects of metformin and vildagliptin in adult rats with insulin resistance induced by a high-fat diet. *Endocrinology* 153, 3878-85.

[269] Apaijai, N.; Chinda, K.; Palee, S.; Chattipakorn, S. and Chattipakorn, N. (2014) Combined vildagliptin and metformin exert better cardioprotection than monotherapy against ischemia-reperfusion injury in obese-insulin resistant rats. *PLoS One* 9, e102374.

[270] Inthachai, T.; Lekawanvijit, S.; Kumfu, S.; Apaijai, N.; Pongkan, W.; Chattipakorn, S.C. and Chattipakorn, N. (2015) Dipeptidyl peptidase-4 inhibitor improves cardiac function by attenuating adverse cardiac remodelling in rats with chronic myocardial infarction. *Exp. Physiol.* 100, 667-79.

[271] Rizzo, M.R.; Barbieri, M.; Boccardi, V.; Angellotti, E.; Marfella, R. and Paolisso, G. (2014) Dipeptidyl peptidase-4 inhibitors have protective effect on cognitive impairment in aged diabetic patients with mild cognitive impairment. *J. Gerontol. A Biol. Sci. Med. Sci.* 69, 1122-31.

[272] Bullinga, J.R.; Alharethi, R.;Schram, M.S.;Bristow, M.R. and Gilbert, E.M. (2005) Changes in heart rate variability are correlated to hemodynamic improvement with chronic carvidilol therapy in heart failure. *J. Card. Fail.* 11, 693-9.

[273] Nerla, R.; Di Franco, A.; Milo, M.; Pitocco, D.; Zaccardi, F.; Tarzia, P.; Sarullo, F.M.; Villano, A.; Russo, G.; Stazi, A.; Ghirlanda, G.; Lanza, G.A. and Crea, F. (2012) Differential effects of heart rate reduction by atenolol or ivabradine on peripheral endothelial function in type 2 diabetic patients. *Heart* 98, 1812-6.

[274] Currie, C.J.; Poole, C.D.; Evans, M.; Peters, J.R. and Morgan, C.L. (2013) Mortality and other important diabetes-related outcomes with insulin vs other antihyperglycemic therapies in type 2 diabetes. *J. Clin. Endocrinol. Metab.* 98, 668-77.

[275] Scirica, B.M.; Bhatt, D.L.; Braunwald, E.; Steg, P.G.; Davidson, J.; Hirshberg, B.; Ohman, P.; Frederich, R.; Wiviott, S.D.; Hoffman, E.B.; Cavender, M.A.; Udell, J.A.; Desai, N.R.; Mosenzon, O.; McGuire, D.K.; Ray, K.K.; Leiter, L.A. and Raz, I. (2013) Saxagliptin and cardiovascular outcomes in patients with type 2 diabetes mellitus. *N. Engl. J. Med.* 369, 1317-26.

[276] Rojas, L.B. and Gomes, M.B. (2013) Metformin: an old but still the best treatment for type 2 diabetes. *Diabetol. Metab. Syndr.* 5:6.

[277] Zinman, B.; Wanner, C.; Lachin, J.M.; Fitchett, D.; Bluhmki, E.; Hantel, S.; Mattheus, M.; Devins, T.; Johansen, O.E.; Woerle, H.J.; Broedl, U.C. and Inzucchi, S.E. (2015) Empagliflozin, cardiovascular outcomes, and mortality in type 2 diabetes. *N. Engl. J. Med.* 373, 2117-28.

[278] Schatz, H. (2015) Erhöhte Sterblichkeit durch Lungenentzündungen und Sepsis unter dem Diabetes-Medikament Saxagliptin? *Medizinische Kurznachrichten der Deutschen Gesellschaft für Endokrinologie*, 2015 Jul 22.

[279] Syed, S.H.; Gosavi, S.; Shami, W.; Bustamante, M.; Farah, Z.; Teleb, M.; Abbas, A.; Said, S. and Mukherjee, D. (2015) A review of sodium glucose co-transporter 2 inhibitors canagliflozin, dapagliflozin and empagliflozin. Cardiovasc. Hematol. *Agents Med. Chem.* 13, 105-12.

[280] Umpierrez, G.E. and Kitabchi, A.E. (2003) Diabetic ketoacidosis: risk factors and management strategies. *Treat. Endocrinol.* 2, 95-108.

[281] Pfeffer, M.A.; Claggett, B.; Diaz, R.; Dickstein, K.; Gerstein, H.C.; Køber, L.V.; Lawson, F.C.; Ping, L.; Wei, X.; Lewis, E.F.; Maggioni, A.P.; McMurray, J.J.; Probstfield, J.L.; Riddle, M.C.; Solomon, S.D. and Tardif, J.C. Lixisenatide in patients with type 2 diabetes and acute coronary syndrome. *N. Engl. J. Med.* 373, 2247-57.

[282] Druschky, A.; Spitzer, A.; Platsch, G.; Claus, D.; Feistel, H.; Druschky, K.; Hilz, M.J. and Neundörfer, B. (1999) Cardiac sympathetic denervation in early stages of amyotrophic lateral sclerosis demonstrated by 123I-MIBG-SPECT. *Acta Neurol. Scand.* 99, 308-14.

[283] Alonso, A.; Huang, X.; Mosley, T.H.; Heiss, G. and Chen, H. (2015) Heart rate variability and the risk of Parkinson disease: The atherosclerosis risk in communities study. *Ann. Neurol.* 77, 877-83.

[284] Mastrocola, C.; Vanacore, N.; Giovani, A.; Locuratolo, N.; Vella, C.; Alessandri, A.; Baratta, L.; Tubani, L. and Meco, G. (1999) Twenty-four-hour heart rate variability to access autonomic function in Parkinson´s disease. *Acta Neurol. Scand.* 99, 245-7.

[285] Palma, J.A.; Urrestarazu, E.; Alegre, M.; Pastor, M.A.; Valencia. M.; Artieda, J. and Iriarte, J. (2013) Cardiac autonomic impairment during sleep is linked with disease severity in Parkinson´s disease. *Clin. Neurophysiol.* 124, 1163-8.

[286] Fang, F.; Wirdefeldt, K.; Jacks, A.; Kamel, F.; Ye, W. and Chen, H. (2012) Infections and non-communicable disease – CNS infections, sepsis and risk of Parkinson´s disease. *Int. J. Epidemiol.* 41, 1042-9.

[287] Matsumoto, H.; Sengoku, R.; Saito, Y.; Kakuta, Y.; Murayama, S. and Imafuku, I. (2014) Sudden death in Parkinson´s disease: a retrospective autopsy study. *J. Neurol. Sci.* 343, 149-52.

[288] Ishizaki, F.; Harada, T.; Yoshinaga, H.; Nakayama, T.; Yamamura, Y. and Nakamura, S. (1996) [Prolonged QTc intervals in Parkinson´s disease – relation to sudden death and autonomic dysfunction]. *No. To. Shinkei* 48, 443-8.

[289] Deguchi, K.; Sasaki, I.; Tsukaguchi, M.; Kamoda, M.; Touge, T.; Takeuchi, H. and Kuriyama, S. (2002) Abnormalities of rate-corrected QT intervals in Parkinson´s disease – a comparison with multiple system atrophy and progressive supranulear palsy. *J. Neurol. Sci.* 199, 31-7.

[290] Ganguli, M. and Lotze, M.T. (2015) Parkinson Disease and Malignant Disease: Minding Cancer's Own Business. *JAMA Oncol.* 1, 641-2.

[291] Ong, E.L.; Goldacre, R. and Goldacre, M. (2014) Differential risks of cancer types in people with Parkinson´s disease: a national record-linkage study. *Eur. J. Cancer* 50, 2456-62.

[292] Agalliu, I.; San Luciano, M.; Mirelman, A.; Giladi, N.; Waro, B.; Aasly, J.; Inzelberg, R.; Hassin-Baer, S.; Friedman, E.; Ruiz-Martinez, J.; Marti-Masso, J.F.; Orr-Urtreger, A.; Bressman, S. and Saunders-Pullmam, R. (2015) Higher frequency of certain cancers in LRRK2 G2019S mutation carriers with Parkinson disease: a pooled analysis. *JAMA Neurol.* 72, 58-65.

[293] Lin PY, Chang SN, Hsiao TH, Huang, B.T.; Lin, C.H. and Yang, P.C. (2015) Association Between Parkinson Disease and Risk of Cancer in Taiwan. *JAMA Oncol.* 1, 633-40.

[294] Franchi, F.; Lazzeri, C.; Barletta, G.; Ianni, L. and Mannelli, M. (2001) Centrally mediated effects of bromocriptine on cardiac sympathovagal balance. *Hypertension* 38, 123-9.

[295] Wang, V.; Chao, T.H.; Hsieh, C.C. and Lin, C.C.; Kao, C.H. (2015) Cancer risks among the users of ergot-derived dopamine agonists for Parkinson´s disease, a nationwide population-based survey. *Parkinsonism Relat. Disord.* 21, 18-22.

[296] Sriranjini, S.J.; Ganesan, M; Datta, K.; Pal, P.K. and Sathyaprabha, T.N. (2011) Effect of a single dose of standard levodopa on cardiac autonomic function in Parkinson´s disease. *Neurol. India* 59, 659-63.

[297] *Meng, L.*; Dunckley, E.D. and Xu, X. (2015) [Effects of a single dose levodopa on heart rate variability in Parkinson´s disease]. *Zhonghua Yi Xue Za Zhi* 95, 493-5.

[298] Weiner, P.; Inzelberg, R.; Davidovich, A.; Nisipeanu, P.; Magadle, R.; Berar-Yanay, N. and Carasso, R.L. (2002) Respiratory muscle performance and the perception of dyspnoe in Parkinson´s disease. *Can. J. Neurol. Sci.* 29, 68-72.

[299] Olsen, J.H.; Tangerud, K.; Wermuth, L.; Frederiksen, K. and Friis, S. (2007) Treatment with levodopa and risk for malignant melanoma. *Mov. Disord.* 22, 1252-7.

[300] Luthra, P.M. and Kumar, J.B. (2012) Plausible improvements for selective targeting of dopamine receptors in therapy of Parkinson's disease. *Mini Rev. Med. Chem.* 12, 1556-64.

[301] Kuno, S. Progress note on Japanese multicenter bromocriptine monotherapy. *Eur. Neurol.* 33 (Suppl. 1), 3-5.

[302] Kim, J.S. and Sohn, Y.H. (2003) Current status of Parkinson's disease treatment in Korea. *Parkinsonism Relat. Disord.* 9 (Suppl. 2), S99-104.

[303] Weissman, A.; Lowenstein, L.; Peleg, A.; Thaler, I. and Zimmer, E.Z. (2006) Power spectral analysis of heart rate variability during the 100-g oral glucose tolerance test in pregnant woman. *Diabetes Care*, 29, 571-574.

[304] Liao, D.; Cai, J.; Brancati, F.L.; Folsom, A.; Barnes, R.W.; Tyroler, H.A. and Heiss, G. (1995) Association of vagal tone with serum insulin,

glucose, and diabetes mellitus – The ARIC Study. *Diabetes Res. Clin. Pract.* 30, 211-221.

[305] Sun, P.; Zhou, K.; Wang, S.; Li, P.; Chen, S.; Lin, G.; Zhao, Y. and Wang, T. (2013) Involvement of MAPK/NF-κB signaling in the activation of the cholinergic anti-inflammatory pathway in experimental colitis by chronic vagus nerve stimulation. *PLoS One* 8, e69424.

[306] Menezes, R.F.; Bergmann, A.; Aguiar, S.S. and Thuler, L.C. (2015) Alcohol consumption and the risk of cancer in Brazil: A study involving 203,506 cancer patients. *Alcohol* 49, 747-51.

[307] Kawaguchi, M.; Kanemaru, A.; Fukushima, T.; Yamamoto, K.; Tanaka, H.; Haruyama, Y.; Itoh, H.; Matsumoto, N.; Kangawa, K.; Nakazato, M. and Kataoka, H. (2015) Ghrelin administration suppresses inflammation-associated colorectal carcinogenesis in mice. *Cancer Sci.* 106, 1130-6.

[308] Fadul, N.; Strasser, F.; Palmer, J.L.; Yusuf, S.W.; Guo, Y.; Li, Z.; Allo, J. and Bruera, E. (2010) The association between autonomic dysfunction and survival in male patients with advanced cancer: a preliminary report. *J. Pain Symptom. Manage.* 39, 283-90.

[309] Chiang, J.K.; Koo, M.; Kuo, TB. and Fu, C.H. (2010) Association between cardiovascular functions and time to death in patients with terminal hepazocellular carcinoma. *J. Pain Symptom. Manage.* 39, 673-9.

[310] Kim, do H.; Kim, J.A.; Choi, Y.S.; Kim, S.H.; Lee, J.Y. and Kim, Y.E. (2010) Heart rate variability and length of survival in hospice cancer patients. *J. Korean Med. Sci.*, 25, 1140-5.

[311] Lahart, I.M.; Metsios, G.S.; Nevill, A.M. and Carmichael, A.R. (2015) Physical activity, risk of death and recurrence in breast cancer survivors: A systematic review and meta-analysis of epidemiological studies. *Acta Oncol.* 54, 635-54.

[312] Chiang, J.K.; Kuo, T.B.; Fu, C.H. Koo M (2013) Predicting 7-day survival using heart rate variability in hospice patients with non-lung cancers. *PLoS One* 8, e69482.

[313] Togo, F. and Takahashi, M. (2009) Heart rate variability in occupational heath – a systematic review. *Ind. Health* 47, 589-602.

[314] Spottiswoode, J. (2005) Hypothesis: Cancer causes and mechanisms. *Positive Health online* 110, http://www.positivehealth.com/article/cancer/hypothesis-cancer-causes-and-mechanisms.

[315] Magnon, C.; Hall, S.J.; Lin, H.J.; Xue, X.; Gerber, L.; Freedland, S.J. and Frenette, P.S. (2013) Autonomic nerve development contributes to prostate cancer progression. *Science* 341, 1236361.

[316] Pedretti, R.F.; Prete, G.; Foreman, R.D.; Adamson, P.B. and Vanoli, E. (2003) Automic modulation during acute myocardial ischemia by low-dose pirenzepine in conscious dogs with a healed myocardial infarction: a comparison with beta-adrenergic blockade. *J. Cardiovasc. Pharmacol.* 41, 671-7.

[317] Velicer, C.M.; Kristal, A. and White, E. (2006) Alcohol use and the risk of prostate cancer: results from the VITAL cohort study. *Nutr. Cancer* 56, 50-6.

[318] Weise, F.; Müller, D.; Krell, D.; Kielstein, V. and Koch, R.D. (1985) Heart rate variability in withdrawing alcoholic patients. *Drug Alcohol Depend.* 16, 85-88.

[319] Rechlin, T.; Orbes, I.; Weis, M. and Kaschka, W.P. (1996) Autonomic cardiac abnormalities in alcohol-dependent patients admitted to a psychiatric department. *Clin. Auton. Res.* 6, 119-22.

[320] Magnon, C. (2015) Role of the autonomic nervous system in tumorigenesis and metastasis. *Mol. Cell. Oncol.* 2, 2.

[321] Li, S.; Sun, Y, and Gao, D. (2013) Role of the nervous system in cancer metastasis (Review) *Oncol. Lett.* 5, 1101-11.

[322] Cole, S.W.; Nagaraja, A.S.; Lutgendorf, S.K.; Green, P.A. and Sood, A.K. (2015) Sympathetic nervous system regulation of the tumor microenvironment. *Nat. Rev. Cancer* 15, 563-72.

[323] Vander Heiden, M.G.; Cantley, L.C. and Thompson, C.B. (2009) Understanding the Warburg Effect: The metabolic requirements of cell proliferation. *Science* 324, 1029-33.

[324] Semenza, G.L. (2008) Tumor metabolsm: cancer cells give and take lactate. *J. Clin. Invest.* 118, 3835-7.

[325] Cuezva, J.M.; Ortega, Á.D.; Willers, I.M.; Sánchez-Cenizo, L.; Aldea, M. and Sánchez-Aragó, M. (2009) *Biochem. Biophys. Acta* 1792, 1145-58.

[326] Held-Warmkessel, J. and Dell, D.D. (2014) Lactic acidosis in patients with cancer. *Clin. J. Oncol. Nurs.* 18, 592-4.

[327] Elhomsy, G.C.; Eranki, V.; Albert, S.G.; Fesler, M.J.; Parker, S.M.; Michael, A.G. and Griffing, G.T. (2012) "Hyper-warburgism, a cause of

asymptomatic hypoglycemia with lactacidosis in a patient with non-Hodgkin´s lymphoma." *J. Clin. Endocrinol. Metab.* 97, 4311-6.

[328] Sonveaux, P.; Végran, F.; Schroeder, T.; Wergin, M.C.; Verrax, J.; Rabbani, Z.N.; De Saedeleer, C.J.; Kennedy, K.M.; Diepart, C.; Jordan, B.F.; Kelley, M.J.; Gallez, B.; Wahl, M.L.; Feron, O. and Dewhirst, M.W. (2008) Targeting lactate-fueled respiration selectively kills hypoxic tumor cells in mice. *J. Clin. Invest.* 118, 3930-42.

[329] Schurr, A.; Payne, R.S.; Miller, J.J. and Rigor, B.M. (1997) Brain lactate is an obligatory aerobic energy substrate for functional recovery after hypoxia: further in vitro validation. *J. Neurochem.* 69, 423-6.

[330] Deligiannis, A.; Kouidi, E. and Tourkantonis, A. (1999) Effects of physical training on heart rate variability in patients on hemodyalysis. *Am. J. Cardiol.* 84, 197-202.

[331] Chen, Y.; Cairns, R.; Papandreou, I.; Koong, A. and Denko, N.C. (2009) Oxygen consumption can regulate the growth of tumors, a new perspective on the Warburg effect. *PLoS One* 4, e7033.

[332] Makino, H.; Noda, K.; Inagaki, Y.; Horie, H.; Osegawa, M.; Kanatsuka, A. and Yoshida, S. (1985) Lactic acidosis and hypoglycemia associated with acute leukemia. *Jpn. J. Med.* 24, 257-62.

[333] Solaini, G.; Baracca, A.; Lenaz, G. and Sgarbi, G. (2010) Hypoxia and mitochondrial oxidative metabolism. *Biochem. Biophys. Acta* 1797, 1171-7.

[334] Nolop, K.B.; Rhodes, C.G.; Brudin, L.H.; Beaney, R.P.; Krausz, T.; Jones, T. and Hughes, J.M. (1987) Glucose utilization in vivo by human pulmonary neoplasms. *Cancer* 60, 2682-9.

[335] Sillos, E.M.; Shenep, J.L.; Burghen, G.A.; Pui, C.H.; Behm, F.G. and Sandlund, J.T. (2001) Lactic acidosis: a metabolic complication of hematologic malignancies: case report and review oft he literature. *Cancer* 92, 2237-46.

[336] Xie, J.; Wu, H.; Dai, C.; Pan, Q.; Ding, Z.; Hu, D.; Ji, B.; Luo, Y. and Hu, X. (2014) Beyond Warburg effect – dual metabolic nature of cancer cells. *Sci. Rep.* 4, 4927.

[337] DeBerardinis, R.J.; Lum, J.J.; Hatzivassiliou, G. and Thompson, C.B. (2008) The biology of cancer: Metabolic reprogramming fuels cell growth and proliferation. *Cell Metabolism* 7, 11-20.

[338] Knuth S (2008) Reaktionen im Bereich des kardio-vaskulären Systems auf Interventionen akuter und chronischer Hypoxie unter normobaren

Bedingungen. Thesis, Deutsche Sporthochschule Köln, http://www. vifasport.de/Dissertationen/2008/Sarah-Knuth.html.

[339] Scalvini, S.; Porta, R.; Zanelli, E.; Volterrani, M.; Vitacca, M.; Pagani. M.; Giordano, A. and Ambrosino, N. (1999) Effects of oxygen on autonomic nervous system dysfunction in patients with chronic obstructive pulmonary disease. *Eur. Respir. J.* 13, 119-24.

[340] Botek, M.; Lrejčí, J.; De Smet, S.; Gába, A. and McKune, A.J. (2015) Heart rate variability and arterial oxygen saturation response during extreme normobaric hypoxia. *Auton. Neurosci.*, 190 40-5.

[341] Liu, X.X.; Lu, L.L.; Zhong, C.F.; Cheng, Z.H.; Yuan, Q. and Ren, H.R. (2001) [Analysis of heart rate variability during acute exposure to hypoxia]. *Space Med. Med. Eng. (Beijing)* 14, 328-31.

[342] Buchheit, M.; Richard, R.; Doutreleau, S.; Lonsdorfer-Wolf, E.; Brandenberger, G. and Simon, C. (2004) Effect of acute hypoxia on heart rate variability at rest and during exercise. *Int. J. Sports Med.* 25, 264-9.

[343] Al Haddad, H.; Mendez-Villanueva, A.; Bourdon, P.C. and Buchheit, M. (2012) Effect of acute hypoxia on post-exercise parasympathetic reactivation in healthy men. *Front. Physiol.* 3, 289.

[344] Boardman, J.P. and Hawdon, J.M. (2015) Hypoglycemia and hypoxic-ischaemic encephalopathy. *Dev. Med. Child Neurol.* 57 (Suppl. 3), 29-33.

[345] Limberg. J.K.; Dube, S.; Kuijpers, M.; Farni, K.E.; Basu, A.; Rizza, R.A.; Curry, T.B.; Basu, R. and Joyner, M.J. (2015) Effect of hypoxia on heart rate variability and baroreflex sensitivity during hypogkycemia in type 1 diabetes mellitus. *Clin. Auton. Res.* 25, 243-50.

[346] Punsoni, M.; Drexler, S.; Palaia, T.; Stevenson, M. and Stecker, M.M. (2015) Acute anoxic changes in peripheral nerve: anatomic and physiologic correlations. *Brain Beh.* 5, e00347.

[347] Abadie, D.; Durrieu, G.; Roussin, A. and Montastruc, J.L. (2013) ["Serious" adverse drug reactions with tramadol: a 2010-2011 pharmacovigilance survey in France]. *Therapie* 68, 77-84.

[348] Fournier, J.P.; Azoulay, L.; Yin, H.; Montastruc, J.L. and Suissa, S. (2015) Tramadol use and the risk of hospitalization for hypoglycemia in patients with noncancer pain. *JAMA Intern. Med. 175*, 186-93.

[349] Faskowitz, A.J.; Kramskiy, V. N. and Pasternak, G.W. (2013) Methadone-induced hypoglycemia. *Cell. Mol. Neurobiol.* 33, 537-42.

[350] Moryl, N.; Pope, J. and Obbens, E. (2013) Hypoglycemia during rapid methadone dose escalation. *J. Opioid Manag.* 9, 29-34.

[351] Vaupel, P, and Mayer, A. (2014) Hypoxia in tumors: pathogenesis-related classification, characterization of hypoxia subtypes, and associated biological and clinical implications. *Adv. Exp. Med. Biol.* 812, 19-24.

[352] Agamanolis, D.P. (2013) Cerebral ischemia and stroke. Hypoxic-ischemic encephalopathy. General Principles, Neuropathology Chapter 2. http://neuropathology-web.org/chapter2/chapter2cCerebralhemorrhage.html.

[353] Coulter, J.A.; McCarthy, H.O.; Xiang, J.; Roedl, W.; Wagner, E.; Robson, T. and Hirst, D.G. (2008) Nitric oxide – A novel therapeutic for cancer. *Nitric Oxide* 19, 192-8.

[354] Singh, S. and Gupta, S.K. (2011) Nitric oxide: role in tumour biology and iNOS/NO-based anticancer therapies. *Cancer Chemother. Pharmacol.* 57, 1211-24.

[355] Rocha, G.Z.; Dias, M.M.; Ropelle, E.R.; Osório-Costa, F.; Rossato, F.A.; Vercesi, A.E.; Saad, M.J. and Carvalheira, J.B. (2011) Metformin amplifies chemotherapy-induced AMPK activation and antitumoral growth. *Clin. Cancer Res.* 17, 3993-4005.

[356] Kankotia, S. and Stacpoole, P.W. (2014) Dichloroacetate and cancer: new home for an orphan drug? *Biochem. Biophys. Acta* 1846, 617-29.

[357] Xie, Q.; Zhang, H.F.; Guo, Y.Z.; Wang, P.Y.; Liu, Z.S.; Gao, H.D. and Xie, W.L. (2015) Combination of Taxol® and dichloroacetate results in synergistically inhibitory effects on Taxol-resistent oral cancer cells under hypoxia. *Mol. Med. Rep.* 11, 2935-40.

[358] Bernsen, H.J.; van der Kogel, A.J.; van Daal, W.A. and Rijken, P.F. (1997) [Vascularization and perfusion of tumors as target in cancer therapy]. *Ned. Tijdschr. Geneeskd.* 141, 364-8.

[359] Fukumura, D.; Kashiwagi, S. and Jain, R.K. (2006) The role of nitric oxide in tumour progression. *Nat. Rev. Cancer* 6, 521-34.

[360] Sonveaux, P.; Jordan, B.F.; Gallez, B. and Feron, O. (2009) Nitric oxide delivery to cancer: why and how? *Eur. J. Cancer* 45, 1352-69.

[361] Chen, Y.; Zhang, S.; Peng, G.; Yu, J.; Liu, T.; Meng, R.; Li, Z.; Zhao, Y. and Wu, G. (2013) Endothelial NO synthase and reactive oxygen species mediated effect of simvastatin on vessel structure and function:

pleiotropic and dose-dependent effect on tumor vascular stabilization. *Int. J. Oncol.* 42, 1325-36.

[362] Batchelor, T.T.; Gerstner, E.R.; Emblem, K.E.; Duda, D.G.; Kalpathy-Cramer, J.; Snuderl, M.; Ancukiewicz, M.; Polaskova, P.; Pinho, M.C.; Jennings, D.; Plotkin, S.R.; Chi, A.S.; Eichler, A.F.; Dietrich, J.; Hochberg, F.H.; Lu-Emersson, C.; Iafrate, A.J.; Ivy, S.P.; Rosen, B.R.; Loeffler, J.S.; Wen, P.Y.; Sorensen, A.G. and Jain, R.K. (2013) Improved tumor oxygenation and survival in glioblastoma patients who show increased blood perfusion after cediranib and chemoradiation. *Proc. Natl. Acad. Sci. USA* 110, 19059-64.

[363] Jordan, B.F. and Sonveaux, P. (2012) Targeting tumor perfusion and oxygenation to improve the outcome of anticancer therapy. *Front. Pharmacol.* 3, 94.

[364] Vallianou, N.G.; Avangelopoulos, A. and Kazazis, C. (2013) Metformin and Cancer. *Rev. Diabet. Stud.* 10, 228-35.

[365] Molfino, A.; Gioia, G.; Fanelli, F.R. and Laviano, A. (2015) Contribution of neuroinflammation to the pathogenesis of cancer cachexia. *Mediators Inflamm.* 2015, 801685.

[366] Uusitalo, A.L.; Laitinen, T.; Väisänen, S.B.; Länsimies, E. and Rauramaa, R. (2002) Effects of endurance training on heart rate and blood pressure variability. *Clin. Physiol. Funct. Imaging* 22, 173-9.

[367] Lira, F.S.; Antunes, B.M.; Seelaender, M. and Neto, J.C. (2015) The therapeutic potential of exercise to treat cachexia. *Curr. Opin. Support Palliat. Care* 9, 317-24.

[368] Laviano, A.; Koverech, A. and Mari, A. (2015) Cachexia: clinical features when inflammation drives malnutrition. *Proc. Nutr. Soc.* 74, 348-54.

[369] Goodwin, M.L.; Gladden, L.B.; Nijsten, M.W. and Jones, K.B. (2015) Lactate and cancer: revisiting the Warburg effect in an era of lactate shuttling. *Front. Nutr.* 1, 27.

[370] Bongaerts, G.P.; van Halteren, H.K.; Verhagen, C.A. and Wagener, D.J. (2006) Cancer cachexia demonstrates the energy impact of gluconeogenesis in human metabolism. *Med. Hypotheses* 67, 1213-22.

[371] Yang, J.C.; Dai, Y.Y.; Wang, L.M.; Xie, Y.B.; Zhou, H.Y. and Li, G.H. (2015) Glycemic variation in tumor patients with total parenteral nutrition. *Chin. Med. J. (Engl.)* 128, 2034-9.

[372] Togni, V.; Ota, C.C.; Folador, A.; Júnior, O.T.; Aikawa, J.; Yamazaki, R.K.; Freitas, F.A.; Longo, R.; Martins, E.F.; Calder, P.C.; Curi, R. and Fernandes, L.C, (2003) Cancer cachexia and tumor growth reduction in Walker 256 tumor-bearing rats supplemented with N-3 polyunsaturated fatty acids for one generation. *Nutr. Cancer* 46, 52-8.

[373] Folador, A.; Hirabara, S.M.; Bonatto, S.J.; Aikawa, J.; Yamazaki, R.K.; Curi, R. and Fernandes, L.C. (2007) Effects of fish oil supplemention for 2 generations on changes in macrophage function induced by Walker 256 cancer cachexia in rats. *Int. J. Cancer* 120, 344-50.

[374] Aoyagi, T.; Terracina, K.P.; Raza, A.; Matsubara, H. and Takabe, K. (2015) Cancer cachexia, mechanism and tratment. *World J. Gastrointest. Oncol.* 7, 17-29.

[375] Yildirir, A.; Kabakci, G.; Yarali, H.; Aybar, F.; Akgul, E.; Bukulmez, O.; Tokgozoglu, L.; Gurgan, T. and Oto, A. (2001) Effects of hormone replacement therapy on heart rate variability in postmenopausal women. *Ann. Noninvasive Electrocardiol.* 6, 280-4.

[376] Soeki, T.; Kishimoto, I.; Schwenke, D.O.; Tokudome, T.; Horio, T.; Yoshida, M.; Hosoda, M. and Kangawa, K. (2008) Ghrelin suppresses cardiac sympathetic activity and prevents early left ventricular remodeling in rats with myocardial infarction. *Am. J. Physiol. Heart Circ. Physiol.* 294, H426-32.

[377] Huda, M.S.; Mani, H.; Dovey, T.; Halford, J.C.; Boyland, E.; Daousi, C.; Wilding, J.P. and Pinkney, J. (2010) Ghrelin inhibits autonomic function in healthy controls, but has no effect on obese and vagotomized subjects. *Clin. Endocrinol. (Oxf.)* 73, 678-85.

[378] Mao, Y.; Tokudome, T.; Otani, K.; Kishimoto, I.; Nakanishi, M.; Hosoda, H.; Miyazato, M. and Kangawa, K. (2012) Ghrelin prevents incidence of malignant arrhythmia after acute myocardial infarction through vagal afferent nerves. *Endocrinology* 153, 3426-34.

[379] Virtanen, I.; Polo, O.; Saaresranta, T.; Kuusela, T.; Polo-Kantola, P. and Ekholm, E. (2004) Medroxyprogesterone improves cardiac autonomic control in postmenopausal women with respiratory insufficiency. *Respir. Med.* 98, 126-33.

[380] Hassoun, E.; Kariya, C. and Williams, F.E. (2005) Dichloroacetate-induced developmental toxicity and production of reactive oxygen species in zebrafish embryos. *J. Biochem. Mol. Toxicol.* 19, 52-8.

[381] Saed, G.M.; Fletcher, N.M.; Jiang, Z.L.; Abu-Soud, H.M. and Diamond, M.P. (2011) Dichloroacetate induces apoptosis of epithelial ovarian cancer cells through a mechanism involving modulation of oxidative stress. *Reprod. Sci.* 18, 1253-61.

[382] Sutendra, G. and Michelakis, E.D. (2013) Pyruvate dehydrogenase kinase as a novel therapeutic target in oncology. *Front. Oncol.* 3, 38.

[383] Ley, S.H.; Sun, Q.; Willett, W.C.; Eliassen, A.H.; Wu, K,; Pan, A.; Grodstein. F. and Hu, F.B. (2014) Associations between red meat intake and biomarkers of inflammation and glucose metabolism in women. *Am. J. Clin. Nutr.* 99, 352-60.

[384] Samraj, A.N.; Pearce, O.M.; Läubli, H.; Crittenden, A.N.; Bergfeld, A.K.; Banda, K.; Gregg, C.J.; Bingman, A.E.; Secrest, P.; Diaz, S.L.; Varki, N.M. and Varki, A. (2015) A red meat-derived glycan promotes inflammation and cancer progression. *Proc. Natl. Acad. Sci. USA* 112, 542-7.

[385] Bouvard, V.; Loomis, D.; Guyton, K.Z.; Grosse, Y.; Ghissassi, F.E.; Benbrahim-Tallaa, L.; Guha, N.; Mattock, H. and Straif, K. (2015) Carcinogenity of consumption of red and processed meat. *Lancet Oncol.* 16, 1599-600.

[386] Montonen, J.; Boeing, H.; Fritsche, A.; Schleicher, E.; Joost, H.G.; Schulze, M.B.; Steffen, A. and Pischon, T. (2013) Consumption of red meat and whole-grain bread in relation to biomarkers of obesity, inflammation, glucose metabolism and oxidative stress. *Eur. J. Nutr.* 52, 337-45.

[387] Anand, P.; Kunnumakkara, A.B.; Sundaram, C.; Harikumar, K.B.; Tharakan, S.T.; Lai, O.S.; Sung, B. and Aggarwal, B.B. (2008) Cancer is a preventable disease that requires major lifestyle changes. *Pharm. Res.* 25, 2097-116.

[388] Zhong, J.; Colicino, E.; Lin, X.; Metha, A.; Kloog, I.; Zaobetti, A.; Byun, H.M.; Bind, M.A.; Cantone, L.; Prada, D.; Tarantini, L.; Trevisi, L.; Sparrow, D.; Vokonas, P.; Schwartz, J. and Baccarelli, A.A. (2015) Cardiac autonomic dysfunction: Particulate air pollution effects are modulated by epigenetic immunoregulation of Toll-like receptor 2 and diatary flavonoid intake. *J. Am. Heart Assoc.* 4, e001423.

[389] Song, M.; Garret, W.S. and Chan, A.T. (2015) Nutients, foods, and colorectal prevention. *Gastroenterology* 148, 1244-60.

[390] Zheng, J.S.; Hu, X.J., Zhao, Y.M.; Yang, J. and Li, D. (2013) Intake of fish and marine n-3 polyunsaturated fatty acids and risks of breastcancer: meta-analysis of data from 21 independent prospective cohort studies. *B.M.J.* 346, f3706.

[391] Park, J.M.; Kwon, S.H.; Han, Y.M.; Hahm, K.B. and Kim, E.H. (2013) Omega-3 polyunsaturated fatty acids as potential chemopreventive agent for gastrointestinal cancer. *J. Cancer Prev.* 18, 201-8.

[392] Khankari, N.K.; Bradshaw, P.T.; Steck, S.E.; He, K.; Olshan, A.F.; Shen, J.; Ahn, J.; Chen, Y.; Ahsan, H.; Terry, M.B.; Teitelbaum, S.L.; Neugut, A.I.; Santella, R.M. and Gammon, M.D. (2015) Polyunsaturated fatty acid interactions and breast cancer incidence: a population-based case-control study on Long Island, New York. *Ann. Epidemiol.*, 2015 Sep 14.

[393] Inoue-Choi, M.; Sinha, R.; Gierach, G.L. and Ward, M.H. (2015) Red and processed meat, nitrite, and heme iron intakes and postmenopausal breast cancer risk in the NIH-AARP Diet and Health Study. *Int. J. Cancer*, 2015 Oct 27.

[394] Jiao, L.; Stolzenberg-Solomon, R.; Zimmerman, T.P.; Duan, Z.; Chen, L.; Kahle, L.; Risch, A.; Subar, A.F.; Cross, A.J.; Hollenbeck, A.; Vlassara, H.; Striker, G. and Sinha, R. (2015) Dietary consumption of advanced glycation end products and pancreatic cancer in the prospective MIH-AARP Diet and Healthy Study. *Am. J. Clin. Nutr.* 101, 126-34.

[395] Chiang, V.S. and Quek, S.Y. (2015) The relationship of red meat with cancer: Effects of thermal processing and related physiological mechanisms. *Crit. Rev. Food Sci. Nutr.*, 2015 Jun 15.

[396] Centritto, F.; Iacoviello, L.; di Giuseppe, R.; De Curtis, A.; Constanzo, S.; Zito, F.; Grino, S.; Siero, S.; Donati, M.B.; de Gaetano, G. and Di Castelnuevo, A. (2009) Dietary patterns, cardiovascular risk factors and C-reactive protein in a healthy Italian population. *Nutr. Metab. Cardiovasc. Dis.* 19, 697-706.

[397] van Woudenbergh, G.J.; Kuijsten, A.K.; Tigcheler, B.; Sijbrands, E.J.; van Rooij, F.J.; Hofman, A.; Witteman, J.C. and Feskens, E.J. (2012) Meat consumption and its association with C-reactive protein and incident type 2 diabetes. The Rotterdam Study. *Diabetes Care* 35, 1499-1505.

[398] N.N. (2015) Bacon, sausages, ham and other processed meats are cancer-causing, red meat probably is too: WHO. http://www.abc.net.au/news/2015-10-27/processed-meats-cause-cancer-says-un-agency/6886882.

[399] Granic, A.; Davies, K.; Adamson, A.; Kirkwood, T.; Hill, T.R.; Siervo, M.; Mathers, J.C. and Jagger, C. (2016) Dietary patterns high in red meat, potato, gravy, and butter are associated with poor cognitive functioning but not with rate of cognitive decline in very old adults. *J. Nutr.* 2016 Jan 6.

[400] Nehlig, A. (2013) The neuroprorective effects of cocao flavanol and its influence on cognitive performance. *Br. J. Pharmacol.* 75, 716-27.

[401] Chew, M.L.; Mulsant, B.H.; Pollock, B.G.; Lehman, M.E.; Greenspan, A.; Mahmoud, R.A.; Kirshner, M.A.; Sorisio, D.A.; Bies, R.R. and Gharabawi, G. (2008) Anticholinergic activity of 107 medications commonly used by older adults. *J. Am. Geriatr. Soc.* 56, 1333-41.

[402] Kaya, D.; Ellidokuz, E.; Onrat, E.; Ellidokuz, H.; Celik, A. and Kilit, C. (2003) The effect of dopamine type-2 receptor blockade on autonomic modulation. *Clin. Auton. Res.*, 13, 275-80.

[403] Neki, N.S.; Singh, R.B. and Rastogi, S.S. (2004) How brain influences neuro-cardiovascular dysfunction. *J. Assoc. Physicians India* 52, 223-30.

[404] Baur, D.M.; Klotsche, J.; Hamnvik, O.P.; Sievers, C.; Pieper, L.; Wittchen, H.U.; Stalla, G.K.; Schmid, R.M.; Kales, S.N. and Mantzoros, C.S. (2011) Type 2 diabetes mellitus and medications for type 2 diabetes mellitus are associated with risk for and mortality from cancer in a German primary care cohort. *Metabolism* 60, 1363-71.

[405] Graber, D.J.; Hickey, W.F.; Stommel, E.W. and Harris, B.T. (2012) Anti-inflammatory efficacy of dexamethasone and Nrf2 activators in the CNS using brain slices as a model of acute unjury. *J. Neuroimmune Pharmacol.* 7, 266-78.

[406] Kontopoulos, A.G.; Athyros, V.G.; Papageorgiou, A.A.; Papadopoulos, G.V.; Avramidis, M.J. and Boudoulas, H. (1996) Effect of quinapril or metoprolol on heart rate variability in post-myocardial infarction patients. *Am. J. Cardiol.* 77, 242-6.

[407] Nousiainen, T.; Vanninen, E.; Jantunen, E.; Remes, J.; Ritanen, E.; Vuolteenaho, O. and Hartikainen, J. (2001) Neuroendocrine changes during the evolution of doxorubicin-induced left ventricular dysfunction in adult lymphoma patients. *Clin. Sci. (Lond.)* 101, 601-7.

[408] Hirvonen, H.E.; Salmi, T.T.; Heinonen, E.; Antila, K.J.; Välimäki, I.A. (1989) Vincristine treatment of acute lymphoblastic leukemia induces transient autonomic cardiopathy. *Cancer*, 64, 801-5.

[409] Ekholm, E.; Rantanen, V.; Bergman, M.; Vesalainen, R.; Antila, K. and Salminen, E. (2000) Docetaxel and autonomic cardiovascular control in anthracycline treated breast cancer patients. *Anticancer Res.* 20, 2045-8.

[410] Casu, M.; Cappi, C.; Patrone, V.; Repetto, E.; Giusti, M.; Minuto, F. and Murialdo, G. (2005) Sympatho-vagal control of heart rate variability in patients treated with suppressive doses of L-thyroxine for thyroid cancer. *Eur. J. Endocrinol.* 152, 819-24.

[411] Hoca, A.; Yildiz, M. and Ozyigit, G. (2012) Evaluation of the effects of mediastinal radiation therapy on autonomic nervous system. *Med. Oncol.* 29, 3581-6.

[412] Mokra, D.; Tonhajzerova, I.; Petraskova, M. and Calkovska, A. (2009) Effects of dexamethasone on cardiovascular functions in acute phase in meconium-injured rabbits. *Pediatr. Int.* 51, 132-7.

[413] Fletcher, N.M.; Awonuga, A.O.; Neubauer, B.R.; Abusamaan, M.S.; Saed, M.G.; Diamond, M.P. and Saed, G.M. (2015) Shifting anaerobic to aerobic modulation of redox balance: potential intervention in the pathogenesis of postoperative adhesions. *Fertil. Steril.* 104, 1022-9.

[414] Xie, J.; Wang, B.S.; Yu. D.H.; Lu, Q.; Ma, J.; Qi, H.; Fang, C. and Chen, H.Z. (2011) Dichloroacetate shifts the metabolism from glycolysis to glucose oxidation and exhibits synergistic growth inhibition with cisplatin in HeLa cells. *Int. J. Oncol.* 38, 409-17.

[415] Lin, C.C.; Yeh, H.H.; Huang, W.L.; Yan, J.J.; Lai, W.W.; Su, W.P.; Chen, H.H. and Su, W.C. (2013) Metfomin enhances cisplatin cytotoxicity by suppressing signal transducer and activator of transcription-3-activity independently of the liver kinase B1-AMP-activated protein kinase pathway. *Am. J. Respir. Cell. Mol. Biol.* 49, 241-50.

[416] Marchiq, I. and Pouysségur, J. (2015) Hypoxia, cancer metabolism and the therapeutic benefit of targeting lactate/H^+ symporters. *J. Mol. Med. (Berl.)*, 2015 Jun 24.

[417] De Couck, M.; van Brummelen, D.; Schallier, D.; De Grève, J. and Gidron, Y. (2013) The relationship between vagal nerve activity and clinical outcomes in prostate and non-small cell lung cacer patients. *Oncol. Rep.* 30, 2435-41.

[418] Guo, Y.; Palmer, J.L.; Strasser, F.; Yusuf, S.W. and Bruera, E. (2013) Heart rate variability as a measure of autonomic dysfunction in men with advanced cancer. *Eur. J. Cancer Care (Engl.)* 22, 612-6.

[419] Kim, K.; Chae, J. and Lee, S. (2015) The role of heart rate variability in advanced non-small-cell lung cancer patients. *J. Palliat.* 31, 103-8.

[420] Holman, A.J. and Ng, E. (2008) Heart rate variability predicts anti-tumor necrosis factor therapy response for inflammatory arthritis. *Auton. Neurosci.* 143, 58-67.

[421] Rossi, S.; Rocchi. C.; Studer, V.; Motta, C.; Lauretti, B.; Germani, G.; Macchiarulo, G.; Marfia, G.A. and Centonze, D. (2015) The autonomic balance predicts cardiac responses after the first dose of fingolimod. *Mult. Scler.* 21, 206-16.

[422] Infusino, F.; Pitocco, D.; Zaccardi, F.; Scavone, G.; Coviello, I.; Nerla, R.; Mollo, R.; Sestito, A.; Di Monaco, A.; Barone, L.; Pisanello, C.; Ghirlanda, G.; Lanza, G.A. and Crea, F. (2010) Low glucose levels are associated with abnormal cardiac sympatho-vagal balance in type 2 diabetic patients with coronary artery disease. *Eur. Rev. Med. Pharmacol. Sci.* 14, 203-207.

[423] Limberg, J.K.; Farni, K.E.; Taylor, J.L.; Dube, S.; Basu, R.; Wehrwein, E.A. and Joyner, M.J. (2014) Autonomic control during acute hypoglycemia in type 1 diabetes mellitus. *Clin. Auton. Res.*, 2014 Sep 27.

[424] Cacciatori, V.; Gemma, M.L.; Bellavere, F.; Castello, R.; De Gregori, M.E.; Zoppini, G.; Thomaseth, K.; Moghetti, P. and Muggeo, M. (2000) Power spectral analysis of heart rate in hypothyroidism. *Eur. J. Endocrinol.* 143, 327-33.

[425] Portella, R.B.; Pedrosa, R.C. Coeli, C.M.; Buescu, A. and Vaisman, M. (2007) Altered cardiovascular vagal responses in nonelderly female patients with subclinical hyperthyroidism and no apparent cardiovascular disease. *Clin. Endocrin. (Oxf.)* 67, 290-4.

[426] Lindsey, J.W.; Haden-Pinneri, K.; Memon, N.B. and Buja, L.M. (2012) Sudden unexpected death on fingolimod. *Mult. Scler.* 18, 1507-8.

[427] Bektaşli, F.; Yildiz ÖK, Segmen, H.; Bolayir, E. and Topaktaş, S. (2009) Heart rate variability in patients with multiple sclerosis. *J. Neurol. Sci.* 26, 271-8.

[428] Mahovic, D.M. and Lakusic, N. (2007) Progressive impairment of autonomic control of heart rate in patients with multiple sclerosis. *Arch. Med. Res.* 38, 322-5.

[429] Tombul, T.; Anlar, O.; Tuncer, M.; Huseyinoglu, N. and Eryonucu, B. (2011) Impaired heart rate variability as a marker of cardiovascular autonomic dysfunction in multiple sclerosis. *Acta Neurol. Belg.* 111, 116-20.

[430] Kappos, L.; Cohen, J.; Collins, W.; de Vera, A.; Zhang-Auberson, L.; Ritter, S.; von Rosenstiel, P. and Francis, G. (2014) Fingolimod in relapsing multiple sclerosis: An integrated analysis of safety findings. *Mult. Scler. Relat. Disord.* 3, 494-504.

[431] Paolicelli, D.; Manni, A.; Direnzo, V.; D´Onghia, M.; Tortorella, C.; Zoccolella, S. and Trojano, M. (2015) Long term cardiac safety and tolerability of fingolimod in multiple sclerosis: A post-marketing study. *J. Clin. Pharmacol.* 55, 1131-6.

[432] Boolani, H.; Shanberg, D.; Chikkam, V. and Lakkireddy, D. (2011) Metformin associated atrial fibrillation – a case report. *JAFIB 4, 3.*

[433] Rolf, L. and Muris, A.H. (2014) Paroxysmal atrial fibrillation after initiation of fingolimod for multiple sclerosis treatment. *Neurology* 82, 1008-9.

[434] Gialafos, E.; Gerakoulis, S.; Grigoriou, A.; Haina, V.; Kilidireas, C.; Stamboulis, E. and Andreadou, E. (2014) Intermittent atrioventricular block following fingolimod initiation. *Case Rep. Neurol. Med.* 2014, 191305.

[435] Azuma, H.; Takahara, S.; Ichimaru, N.; Wang, J.D.; Itoh, Y.; Otsuki, Y.; Morimoto, J.; Fukui, R.; Hoshiga, M.; Ishihara, T.; Nonomura, N.; Suzuki, S.; Okuyama, A. and Katsuoka, Y. (2002) Marked prevention of tumor growth and metastasis by a novel immunosuppressive agent, FTY720, in mouse breast cancer models. *Cancer Res.* 62, 1410-9.

[436] Li, C.X.; Shao, Y.; Ng, K.T.; Liu, X.B.; Ling, C.C.; Ma, Y.Y.; Geng, W.; Fan, S.T.; Lo, C.M. and Man, K. (2012) FTY720 suppresses liver tumor metastasis by reducing the population of circulating endothelial progenitor cells. *PLoS One* 7, e32380.

[437] Simula, S.; Laitinen, T.; Laitinen, T.M.; Tarkiainen, T.; Hartikainen, P. and Hartikainen, J.E. (2015) Effect of fingolimod on cardiac autonomic regulation in patients with multiple sclerosis. *Mult. Scler.*, 2015 Sep 11.

[438] Gonzalez-Cabrera, P.J.; Brown, S.; Studer, S.M. and Rosen, H. (2014) S1P signaling: new therapies and opportunities. *F1000Prime Rep.* 6, 109.

[439] Subel, A.M. and Cohen, J.A. (2015) Sphingosine 1-phosphate receptor modulators in multiple sclerosis. *CNS Drugs* 29, 565-75.

[440] Subei, A.M. and Cohen, J.A. (2015) Sphingosine 1-phosphate receptor modulators in multiple sclerosis. *CNS Drugs* 29, 565-75.

[441] Brossard, P.; Derendorf, H.; Xu, J.; Maatouk, H.; Halabi, A. and Dingemanse, J. (2013) Pharmacokinetics and pharmacodynamics of ponesimod, selective S1P1 receptor modulator, in the first-in-human study. *Br. J. Clin. Pharmacol.* 76, 88-96.

[442] Rey, M.; Hess, P.; Clozel, M.; Delahaye, S.; Gatfield, J.; Nayler, O. and Steiner, B. (2013) Desensification by progressive up-titration prevents first-dose effects on the heart: guinea pig study with ponesimod, a selective S1P1 receptor modulator. *PLoS One* 8, e74285.

[443] Hoch, M.; D´Ambrosio, D.; Wilbraham, D.; Brossard, P. and Dingemanse, J. (2014) Clinical pharmacology of ponesimod, a selective S1P1 receptor modulator, after uptitration to supratherapeutic doses in healthy subjects. *Eur. J. Pharm. Sci.* 63, 147-53.

[444] Scherz. M.W.; Brossard, P.; D´Ambrosio, D.; Ipek, M. and Dingermanse, J. (2015) Three different up-titration regimes of ponesimod, a S1P1 receptor modulator, in healthy subjects. *J. Clin. Pharmacol.* 55, 688-97.

[445] Naruszewicz, M.; Daniewski, M.; Nowicka, G. and Kozlowska-Wojciechowska, M. (2003) Trans-unsaturated fatty acids and acrylamide in food as potential atherosclerosis progression factors. Based on own studies. *Acta Microbiol. Pol.* 52 (Suppl.), 75-81.

[446] Virk-Baker, M.K.; Nagy, T.R.; Barnes, S. and Groopman, J. (2014) Dietary acrylamide and human cancer: A systematic review of literature. *Nutr. Cancer* 66, 774-90.

[447] Lajous, M.; Boutron-Ruault, M.C.; Fabre, A.; Clavel-Chapelon, F. and Romieu, I. (2008) Carbohydrate intake, glycemic index, glycemic load, and risk of postmenopausal breast cancer in a prospective study of French women. *Am. J. Clin. Nutr.* 87, 1384-91.

[448] Nagle, C.M.; Kolahdooz, F.; Ibiebele, T.I.; Olsen, C.M.; Lahmann, P.H.; Green, A.C. and Webb, P.M. (2011) Carbohydrate intake, glycemic

load, glycemic index, and risk of ovarian cancer. *Ann. Oncol.* 22, 1332-8.

[449] Qurrat-ul-Ain and Khan, S.A. (2015) Artificial sweeteners: safe or unsafe? *J. Pak. Med. Assoc.* 65, 225-7.

[450] Graber, D.J.; Hickey, W.F.; Stommel, E.W. and Harris, B.T. (2012) Anti-inflammatory efficacy of dexamethasone and Nrf2 activators in the CNS using brain slices as a model of acute unjury. *J. Neuroimmune Pharmacol.* 7, 266-78.

[451] Lee, D.H.; Gold, R. and Linker, R.A. (2012) Mechanisms of oxidative damage in multiple sclerosis and neurodegenerative diseases: therapeutic modulation via fumaric acid esters. *Int. J. Mol. Sci.* 13, 11783-803.

[452] Seidel, P. and Roth, M. (2013) Anti-inflammatory dimethylfumarate: a potential new therapy for asthma? *Mediators Inflamm.* 2013, 875403.

[453] Arnold, P.; Mojumder, D.; Detoledo, J.; Lucius, R. and Wilms, H. (2014) Pathophysiological processes in multiple sclerosis: focus on nuclear factor erythroid-2-related factor 2 and emerging pathways. *Clin. Pharmacol.* 6, 35-42.

[454] Šilhavý, J.; Zidek, V.; Mlejnek, P.; Landa, V.; Šimáková, M.; Strnad, H.; Oliyarnyk, O.; Škop, V.; Kazdová, L.; Kurtz, T. and Pravenec, M. (2014) Fumaric acid esters can block pro-inflammatory actions of human spontaneously hypertensive rats. *PLoS One* 9, e101906.

[455] Jing, X.; Shi, H.; Zhang, C.; Ren, M.; Han, M.; Wei, X.; Zhang, X. and Lou, H. (2015) Dimethyl fumarate attenuates 6-OHDH-induced neurotoxicity in SH-SY5Y cells and in animal model of Parkinson´s disease by enhancing Nrf2 activity. *Neuroscience* 286, 131-40.

[456] Iniaghe, L.O.; Krafft, P.R.; Klebe, D.W.; Omogbai, E.K.; Zhang, J.H. and Tang, J. (2015) Dimethyl fumarate confers neuroprotection by casein kinase 2 phosphorylation of Nrf2 in murine intracerebral hemorrhage. *Neurobiol. Dis.* 82, 349-58.

[457] Chen, H.; Assmann, J.C.; Krenz, A.; Rahman, M.; Grimm, M.; Karsten, C.M.; Köhl, J.; Offermanns, S.; Wettschureck, N. and Schwaninger, M. (2014) Hydroxycarboxylic acid receptor 2 mediates dimethyl fumarate´s protective effect in EAE. *J. Clin. Invest.* 124, 2188-92.

[458] Tsubaki, M.; Ogawa, N.; Takeda, T.; Sakamoto, K.; Shimaoka, H.; Fujita, A.; Itoh, T.; Imano, M.; Satou, T. and Nishida, S. (2014) Dimethyl fumarate induces apoptosis of hematopoietic tumor cells via

inhibition of NF-κB nuclear translocation and down-regulation of Bcl-xL and XIAP. *Biomed. Pharmacother.* 68, 999-1005.

[459] Xie, X.; Zhao, Y.; Ma, C.Y.; Xu, X.M.; Zhang, Y.Q.; Wang, C.G.; Jin, J.; Shen, X.; Gao, J.L.; Li, J.L.; Sun, Z.J. and Dong, D.L. (2015) Dimethyl fumarate induces necroptosis in colon cancer cells through GSH depletion/ROS increase/MAPKs activation pathway. *Br. J. Pharmacol.* 172, 3929-43.

[460] Chen, A.F. and Kirsner, R.S. (2011) Mechanisms of grug action: The potential of dimethylfumarate for treatment of neoplasms. *J. Invest. Dermatol.* 131, 1181.

[461] Elmståhl, S.; Petersson, M.; Lilja, B.; Samuelsson, S.M.; Rosén, I. and Bjunö, L. (1992) Autonomic cardiovascular responses to tilting in patients with Alzheimer´s sisease and in healthy elderly women. *Age Ageing* 21, 301-7.

[462] McLaren, A.T.; Allen, J.; Murray, M.; Ballard, C.G. and Kenny, R.A. (2003) Cardiovascular effects of donepezil in patients with dementia. Dement. *Geriatr. Cogn. Disord.* 15, 183-8.

[463] Masuda, Y. and Kawamura, A. (2003) Acetylcholinesterase inhibitor (donepezil hydrochloride) reduces heart rate variability. *J. Cardiovasc. Pharmacol.* 41 (Suppl. 1), S67-71.

[464] Siepmann, M.; Mück, A.; Engel, S.; Rupprecht, R. and Mück-Weymann, M. (2006) The influence of rivastigmine and donepezil on heart rate variabiliy in patients with Alzheimer´s disease. *German J. Psychiatry* 9, 133-5.

[465] Handa, T.; Katare, R.G.; Kakinuma, Y.; Arikawa, M.; Ando, M.; Sasaguri, S.; Yamasaki, F. and Sato, T. (2009) Anti-Alzheimer´s drug, donepezil, markedly improves long-term survival after chronic heart failure in mice. *J. Card. Fail.* 15, 805-11.

[466] Li, M.; Zheng, C.; Kawada, T.; Inagaki, M.; Uemura, K.; Shishido, T. and Sugimachi, M. (2013) Donepezil markedly improves long-term survival in rats with chronic heart failure after extensive myocardial infarction. *Circ. J.* 77, 2519-25.

[467] Monacelli, F. and Rosa, G. (2014) Cholinesterase inhibitors: cardioprotection in Alzheimer´s disease. *J. Alzheimers Dis.* 42, 1071-7.

[468] Giubilei, F.; Strano, S.; Imbimbo, B.P.; Tisei, P.; Calcagnini, G.; Lino, S.; Frontoni, M.; Santini, M. and Fieschi, C. (1998) Cardiac autonomic

dysfunction in patients with Alzheimer disease: possible pathogenic mechanisms. *Alzheimer Dis. Assoc. Disord.* 12, 356-61.

[469] da Costa Dias. F.L.; Ferreira Lisboa da Silva, R.M.; de Moraes, E.N. and Caramelli, P. (2013) Cholinesterase inhibitors modulate autonomic function in patients with Alzheimer´s disease and mixed sementia. *Curr. Alzmeimer Res.* 10, 376-81.

[470] Shifrin, H.; Nadler-Milbauer, M.; Shoham, S. and Weinstock, M. (2013) Rivastigmine alleviates experimentally induced colitis in mice and rats by acting at central and peripheral sites to modulate immune responses. *PLoS One* 8, e57668.

[471] Astiz, M.; de Alaniz, M.J. and Marra, C.A. (2012) The oxidative damage and inflammation caused by pesticides are reverted by lipoic acid in rat brain. *Neurochem. Int.* 61, 1231-41.

[472] Kim, Y.H.; Lee, J.H.; Hong, C.K.; Cho, K.W.; Park, Y.H.; Kim, Y.W. and Hwang, S.Y. (2014) Heart rate-corrected QT interval predicts mortality in glyphosate-surfactant herbicide-poisoned patients. *Am. J. Emerg. Med.* 32, 203-7.

[473] Kumar, S.; Khodoun, M.; Kettleson, E.M.; McKnight, C.; Grinshpun, S.A. and Adhikari, A. (2014) Glyphosate-rich air samples induce IL-33, TSLP and generate IL-13 dependent airway inflammation. *Toxicology* 325, 42-51.

[474] Bradberry, S.M.; Proudfoot, A.T. and Vale, J.A. (2004) Glyphosate poisoning. *Toxicol. Rev.*, 23, 159-67.

[475] McNamara, K. and Isbister, G. K. (2015) Hyperlactataemia and clinical severity of acute metformin overdose. *Intern. Med. J.* 45, 402-8.

[476] Talla, V. and Veerareddy, P.R. (2011) Oxidative stress induced by fluoroquinolones on treatment for complicated urinary tract infections in Indian patients. *J. Young Pharm.* 3, 304-309.

[477] Thiyagarajan, R.; Subramanian, S.K.; Sampath, N.; Madanmohan Trakoo, Pal, P.; Bobby, Z.; Paneerselvam, S. and Das, A.K. (2012) Association between cardiac autonomic function, oxidative stress and inflammatory response in impaired fasting glucose subjects: cross sectional study. *PLoS One* 7, e41889.

[478] Jankowska, E.A.; Ponikoweski, P.; Piepoli, M.F.; Banasiak, W.; Anker, S.D. and Poole-Wilson, P.A. (2006) Autonomic imbalance and immune activation in chronic heart failure – pathophysiological links. *Cardiovasc. Res.* 70, 434-45.

[479] Tracey, K.J. (2007) Physiology and immunology oft he cholinergic antiinflammatory pathway. *J. Clin. Invest.* 117, 289-96.

[480] Hall, S.; Kumaria, A. and Belli, A. (2014) The role of vagus nerve overactivity in nthe increased incidence of pneumonia following traumatic brain injury. *Br. J. Neurosurg.* 28, 181-6.

[481] Ahmad, S.; Ramsay, T.; Huebsch, L.; Flanagan, S.; McDiarmid, S.; Batkin, I.; McIntyre, L.; Sundaresan, S.R.; Maziak, D.E.; Shamji, F.M.; Hebert, P.; Fergusson, D.; Tinmouth, A. and Seely, A.J. (2009) Contnuous multi-parameter heart rate variability analysis heralds onset of sepsis in adults. *PLoS One* 4, e6642.

[482] Rao, R. (2009) Endoxemia and gut barrier dysfunction in alcoholic liver disease. Hepatology, 50, 638-644.

[483] Wu, S.; Deng, F.; Niu, J.; Huang, Q.; Liu, Y. and Guo, X. (2008) Association of heart rate variability in taxi drivers with marked changes in particulate air pollution in Beijing in 2008. *Environ. Health Perspect.* 118, 87-91.

[484] Hemmingsen, J.G.; Rissler, J.; Lykkesfeldt, J.; Sallsten, G.; Kristiansen, J.; Møller, P.P. and Loft, S. (2015) Controlled exposure to particulate matter from urban street air is associated with decreased vasodilatation and heart rate variability in overweigth and older adults. *Part. Fibre Toxicol.* 12, 6.

[485] Leeka, J.; Schwartz, B.G. and Kloner, R.A. (2010) Sporting events affect spectators´ cardiovascular mortality: It is not just a game. *Am. J. Med.* 123, 972-7.

[486] Mohapatra, S.P.; Nikolova, I. and Mitchell, A. (2007) Managing mercury in the great lakes: an analytical review of abatement policies. *J. Environ. Manage.* 83, 80-92.

[487] Murata, K.; Grandjean, P. and Dakeishi, M. (2007) Neurophysiological evidence of methylmercury neurotoxicity. *Am. J. Ind. Med.* 50, 765-71.

[488] Valera, B.; Dewailly, E. and Poirier, P. (2008) Cardiac autonomic activity and blood pressure among Nunavik Inuit adults exposed to environmentalmercury: a cross-sectional study. *Environ. Health* 7, 29.

[489] Holt, S.; Schmiedl, S. and Thürmann, P.A. (2010) Potentially inappropriate medications in the elderly: the PRISCUS list. *Dtsch. Arztebl. Int.* 107, 543-51.

[490] Ahmad, S.; Tejuja, A.; Newman, K.D.; Zarychanski, R. and Seely, A.J. (2009) Clinical review: A review and analysis of heart rate variability and diagnosis and prognosis of infection. *Crit. Care* 13, 232.

[491] Fairchild, K.D.; Schelonka, R.L.; Kaufman, D.A.; Carlo, W.A.; Kattwinkel, J.; Porcelli, P.J.; Navarette, C.T.; Bancalari, E.; Aschner, J.L.; Walker, M.W.; Perez, J.A.; Palmer, C.; Lake, D.E.; O´Shea, T.M. and Moorman, J.R. (2013) Septicemia mortality reduction in neonates in a heart rate characteristics monitoring trial. *Pediatr. Res.* 74, 570-5.

[492] Nagaoka, T.; Takahashi, A.; Sato, E.; Izumi, N.; Hein, T.W.; Kuo, L. and Yoshida, A. (2006) Effect of systemic administration of simvastatin on retinal circulation. *Arch. Ophthalmol.* 124, 6665-70.

[493] Stein, J.D.; Newman-Casey, P.A.; Talwar, N.; Nan, B.; Richards, J.E. and Musch, D.C. (2012) The relationship between statin use and open-angle glaucoma. *Ophthalmology* 119, 2074-81.

[494] Chrysostomou, V.; Kezic, J.M.; Trounce, I.A. and Crowston, J.G. (2014) Forced exercise protects the aged optic nerve against intraocular pressure injury. *Neurobiol. Aging* 35, 1722-5.

[495] Castro, E.F.; Mostarda, C.T.; Rodrigues, B.; Moraes-Silva, I.C.; Feriani, D.J.; De Angelis, K.; and Irigoyen, M.C. (2015) Exercise training prevents increased intraocular pressure and sympathetic vascular modulation in an experimental model of metabolic syndrome. *Braz. J. Med. Biol. Res.* 48, 332-8.

[496] Goulopoulou, S.; Baynard, T.; Franklin, R.M.; Fernhall, B.; Carhart, R. Jr.; Weinstock. R. and Kanaley, J.A. (2010) Exercise training improves cardiovascular autonomic modulation in response to glucose ingestion in obese adults with and without type 2 diabetes mellitus. *Metabolism* 59, 901-10.

[497] Deo, S.H.; Fisher, J.P.; Vianna, L.C.; Kim, A.; Chockalingham, A.; Zimmerman, M.C.; Zucker, I.H. and Fadel, P.J. (2012) Statin therapy lowers muscle sympathetic nerve activity and oxidative stress in patients with heart failure. *Am. J. Physiol. Heart Circ. Physiol.* 303, H377-85.

[498] Millar, P.J. and Floras J.S. (2014) Statins and autonomic nervous system. *Clin. Sci. (Lond.)* 126, 401-15.

[499] Routledge, F.S.; Campbell, T.S.; McFetridge-Durdle, J.A. and Bacon, S.L. (2010) Improvements in heart rate variability with exercise therapy. *Can. J. Cardiol.* 26, 303-12.

[500] Sá, J.C.; Costa, E.C.; da Silva, E.; Tamburús, N.Y.; Porta, A.; Medeiros, L.F.; Lemos, T.M.; Soares, E.M. and Azevedo, G.D. (2015) Aerobic exercise improves cardiac autonomic modulation in women with polycystic ovary syndrome. *Int. J. Cardiol.* 202, 356-61.

[501] Laufs, U.; Scharnagl, H.; Halle, M.; Windler, E.; Endres, M. and März, W. (2015) [Treatment options for statin-associated muscle symptoms]. *Dtsch. Arztebl. Int.* 112, 748-55.

[502] Pursnani, A.; Massaro, J.M.; D'Agostino, R.B. Sr.;, O'Donnell, C.J. and Hoffmann, U. (2015) Guideline-based statin eligibility, coronary artery calcification, and cardiovascular events. *JAMA* 314, 134-41.

[503] Saito, I.; Hitsumoto, S.; Maruyama, K.; Eguchi, E.; Kato, T.; Okamoto, A.; Kawamura, R.; Takata, Y.; Nishida, W.; Nishimiya, T.; Onuma, H.; Osawa, H. and Tanigawa, T. (2015) Impact of heart rate variability on C-reactive protein concentrations in Japanese adult nonsmokers: The Toon Health Study. *Atherosclerosis* 244, 79-85.

[504] Schroeder, E.B.; Chambless, L.E.; Liao, D.; Prineas, R.J. and Evans, G.W.; Rosamond, W.D. and Heiss, G. (2005) Diabetes, glucose, insulin, and heart rate variability. The Atherosclerosis Risk in Communities (ARIC) study. *Diabetes Care* 28, 668-674.

[505] Brasileiro-Santos, M.S.; Barreto-Filho, J.A.; Santos, R.D.; Chacra, A.P.; Sangaleti, C.T.; Alvez, G.; Bezerra, O.C.; Bortoloto, L.A.; Irigoyen, M.C. and Consolim-Colombo, F.M. (2013) Statin restores cardiac autonomic response to acute hypoxia in hypercholesterinaemia. *Eur. J. Clin. Invest.* 43, 1291-8.

[506] Al-Khaled. M.; Matthis, C. and Eggers, J. (2014) Statin use in patients with acute ischemic stroke. *Int. J. Stroke* 9, 597-601.

[507] Chen, C.H.; Huang, P.W.; Tang, S.C.; Shieh, J.S.; Lai, D.M.; Wu, A.Y. and Jeng, J.S. (2015) Complexity of Heart Rate Variability Can Predict Stroke-In-Evolution in Acute Ischemic Stroke Patients. *Sci. Rep.* 5, 17552.

[508] Huang, L.Y.; Lin, W.S.; Lin, W.Y.; Cheng, C.C.; Cheng, S.M. and Tsai, T.N. (2013) Torsade de pointes indicates early neurologic damage in acute ischemic stroke. *Am. J. Emerg. Med.* 31, 1719.e5-7.

[509] Lederman, Y.S.; Balucani, C.; Lazar, J.; Steinberg, L.; Gugger, J. and Levine, S.R. (2014) Relationship between QT interval dispersion in acute stroke and stroke prognosis: a systematic review. *J. Stroke Cerebrovasc. Dis.* 23, 2467-78.

[510] Vrtovec, B.; Okrajsek, R.; Golicnik, A.; Ferjan, M.; Starc, V. and Radovancevic, B. (2005) Atorvastatin therapy increases heart rate variability, decreases QT variability, and shortens QTc interval duration in patients with advanced chronic heart failure. *J. Card. Fail.* 11, 684-90.

[511] Xie, R.Q.; Cui, W.; Liu, F.; Yang, C.; Pei, W.N. and Lu, J.C. (2010) Statin therapy shortens QTc, QTcd, and improves cardiac function in patients with chronic heart failure. *Int. J. Cardiol.* 140, 255-7.

[512] Christiansen, C.F.; Christiansen, S.; Farkas, D.K.; Miret, M.; Sørensen, H.T. and Pedersen, I. (2010) Risk of arterial cardiovascular diseases in patients with multiple sclerosis: a population-based cohort study. *Neuroepidemiology* 35, 267-74.

[513] DeGiorgio, C.M.; Miller, P.; Meymandi, S.; Chin, A.; Epps, J.; Gordon, S.; Gornbein, J. and Harper, R.M. (2010) RMSSD, a measure of vagus-mediated heart rate variability, is associated with risk factors for SUDEP: the SUDEP-7 inventory. *Epilepsy Behav.* 19, 78-81.

[514] Cygankiewicz, I. and Zareba, W. (2013) Heart rate variability. Handb. *Clin. Neurol.*, 117, 379-93.

[515] Jadidi, E.; Mohammadi, M. and Moradi, T. (2013) High risk of cardiovascular diseases after diagnosis of multiple sclerosis. *Mult. Scler.* 19, 1336-40.

[516] Roshanisefat, H.; Bahmanyar, S.; Hillert, J.; Olsson, T. and Montgomery, S. (2014) Multiple sclerosis clinical course and cardiovascular disease risk – Swedish cohort study. *Eur. J. Neurol.* 21, 1353-e88.

[517] Na, K.S.; Lee, N.Y.; Park, S.H. and Park, C.K. (2010) Autonomic dysfunction in normal tension glaucoma: the short-term heart rate variability analysis. *J. Glaucoma* 19, 377-81.

[518] Wierzbowska, J.; Wierzbowski, R.; Stankiewicz, A.; Siesky, B. and Harris, A. (2012) Cardiac autonomic dysfunction in patients with normal tension glaucoma: 24-h heart rate and blood pressure variability analysis. *Br. J. Ophthalmol.* 96, 624-8.

[519] DeCastro, D.K.; Punjabi, O.S.; Bostrom, A.G.; Stamper, R.L.; Lietman, T.M.; Ray, K. and Lin, S.C. (2007) Effect of statin drugs and aspirin on progression in open-angle glaucoma suspects using confocal scanning laser ophthalmoscopy. *Clin. Experiment. Ophthalmol.* 35, 506-13.

[520] Marcus, M.W.; Müskens, R.P.; Ramdas, W.D.; Wolfs, R.C.; De Jong, P.T.; Vingerling, J.R.; Hofman, A.; Stricker, B.H. and Jansonius, N. M. (2012) Cholesterol-lowering drugs and incident open-angle glaucoma: a population-based cohort study. *PLoS One* 7: e29724.

[521] Broekmans, W.M.; Vink, A.A.; Boelsma, E.; Klöpping-Ketelaars, W.A.; Tijburg, L.B.; van't Veer, P.; van Poppel, G. and Kardinaal, A.F. (2003) Determinants of skin sensitivity to solar irradiation. *Eur. J. Clin. Nutr.* 57, 1222-9.

[522] Thomas-Ahner, J.M.; Wulff, B.C.; Tober, K.L.; Kusewitt, D.F.; Riggenbach, J.A. and Oberyszyn, T.M. (2007) Gender differences in UVB-induced skin carcinogenesis, inflammation, and DNA damage. *Cancer Res.* 67, 3468-74.

[523] Offner, P.J., Moore, E.E., Biffl, W.L. (1999) Male gender is a risk factor for major infections after surgery. *Arch. Surg. 134,* 935-938.

[524] Bone, R.C. (1992) Toward an epidemiology and natural history of SIRS (systemic inflammatory response syndrome). *JAMA* 268, 3452-3455.

[525] Suefke, S., Djonlagic, H., Kibbel, T. (2012) [Severe bacterial infection: Increased mortality in elderly women with low body weight taking drugs prolonging the QTc interval]. *Med. Klin. Intensivmed. Notfmed.* 107, 275-284.

[526] Le Gal, K.; Ibrahim, M.X.; Wiel, C.; Sayin, V.I.; Akula, M.K.; Karlsson, C.; Dalin, M.G.; Akyürek, L.M.; Lindahl, P.; Nilsson, J. and Bergo, M.O. (2015) Antioxidants can increase melanoma metastasis in mice. *Sci. Transl. Med.* 7, 308re8.

[527] Pal, G.K.; Adithan, C.; Ananthanarayanan, PH.; Pal, P.; Nanda, N.; Thiyagarajan, D.; Syamsunderkiran, A.N.; Lalitha, V. and Dutta, T.K. (2013) Association of sympathovagal imbalance with cardiovascular risks in young prehypertensives. *Am. J. Cardiol.* 112, 1757-62.

[528] Pal, G.K.; Adithan, C.; Ananthanarayanan, P.H.; Pal, P.; Nanda, N.; Durgadevi, T.; Lalitha, V.; Syamsunder, A.N. and Dutta, T.K. (2013) Sympathovagal imbalance contributes to prehypertension status and cardiovascular risks attributed by insulin resistance, inflammation, dyslipidemia and oxidative stress in first degree relatives of type 2 diabetics. *PLoS One* 8, e78072.

[529] Holmes, M.D. and Chen, W.Y. (2012) Hiding in plain view: the potential for commonly used drugs to reduce breast cancer mortality. *Breast Cancer Res.* 14, 216.

[530] Harbaugh, M.P.; Manuck, S.B.; Jennings. J.R.; Conklin, S.M.; Yao, J.K. and Muldoon, M.F. (2013) Long-chain, n-3 fatty acids and physical activity – independent and interactive associations with cardiac autonomic control. *Int. J. Cardiol.* 167, 2102-7.

[531] 116. Deutscher Ärztetag (2013) Ärztetags-Drucksache Nr. VI - 89, http://www.bundesaerztekammer.de/arzt2013/media/applications/EVI89 .pdf.

[532] Klemperer, D. (2015) [Patient involvement as a means to improving care quality]. *Dtsch. Arztebl. Int.* 112, 663-4.

[533] Kanz, R.; Vukovich, T.; Vormittag, R.; Dunkler, D.; Ay, C.; Thaler, J.; Haselböck, J.; Scheithauer, W.; Zielinski, C. and Pabinger, I. (2011) Thrombosis risk and survival in cancer patients with elevated C-reactive protein. *J. Thromb. Haemost.* 9, 57-63.

[534] Miles, JM.; Rule, A.D. and Borlaug, B.A. (2014) Use of metformin in diseases of aging. *Curr. Diab. Rep.* 14, 490.

[535] Hansen, A.L.; Johnsen, B.H.; Sollers, J.J. 3rd; Stenvik, K. and Thayer, J.F. (2004) Heart rate variability and its relation to prefrontal cognitive function effects of training and detraining. *Eur. J. Appl. Physiol.* 93, 263-72.

[536] Hansen, A.L.; Johnsen, B.H. and Thayer, J.F. (2009) Relationship between heart rate variability and cognitive function during threat of shock. *Anxiety Stress Coping* 22, 77-89.

[537] Sun, L.; Chen, R.; Wang, J.; Zhang, Y.; Lin, J.; Peng, W. and Liu, C. (2014) [Association between inflammation and cognitive function and effects of continuous positive airway pressure treatment in obstructive sleep apnea hypopnea sysndrome]. *Zhonghua Yi Xue Za Zhi* 94, 3483-7.

[538] Matei. D.; Popescu, C.D.; Ignat, B. and Matei, R. (2013) Autonomic dysfunction in type 2 diabetes with and without vascular dementia. *J. Neurol. Sci.* 325, 6-9.

[539] N.N. (2016) Kein unausweichliches Schicksal: Das Krebsrisiko lässt sich senken. http://www.gmx.net/magazine/gesundheit/unausweichliches -schicksal-krebsrisiko-laesst-31316064.

[540] Hampel, R.; Breitner, S.; Schneider, A.; Zareba, W.; Kraus, U.; Cyrys, J.; Geruschkat, U.; Belcredi, P.; Müller, M.; Wichmann, H.E. and Peters, A. (2012) Acute air pollution effects on heart rate variability are modyfied by SNPs involved in cardiac rhythm in individuals with diabetes or impaired glucose tolerance. *Environ. Res.* 112, 177-85.

[541] Ramos-Bonilla, J.P.; Breysse, P.N.; Dominici, F.; Geyh, A. and Tankersley, C.G. (2010) Ambient air pollution alters heart rate regulation in aged mice. *Inh. Toxicol.* 22, 330-9.

[542] Zannas, A.S., Arloth, J.; Carillo-Roa, T.; Iurato, S.; Röh, S.; Ressler, K.J.; Nemeroff, C.B.; Smith, A.K.; Bradley, B.; Heim, C.; Menke, A.; Lange, J.F.; Brückl, T.; Ising, M.; Wray, N.R.; Erhardt, A.; Binder E.B. and Metha, D. (2015) Lifetime stress accelerates epigenetic aging in an urban, African American cohort: relevance of glucocorticoid signaling. *Genome Biol.* 16, 266.

[543] Togo, F. and Takahashi, M. (2009) Heart rate variability in occupational heath – a systematic review. *Ind. Health* 47, 589-602.

[544] Jaiswal, M.; Urbina, E.M.; Wadwa, R.P.; Talton, J.W.; D´Agostino, R.B. Jr.; Hamman, R.F.; Fingerlin, T.E.; Daniels, S.R.; Marcovina, S.M.; Dolan, L.M. and Dabelea, D. (2013) Reduced heart rate variability is associated with increased arterial stiffness in youth with type 1 diabetes: the SEARCH CVD study. *Diabetes Care* 36, 2351-8.

[545] Chen, Q.; Chiheb, S.; Fysekidis, M.; Jaber, Y.; Brahimi, M.; Nguyen, M.T.; Millasseau, S.; Cosson, E. and Valensi, P. (2015) Arterila stiffness is elevated in normotensive type 2 diabetic patients with peripheral neuropathy. *Nutr. Metab. Cardiovasc. Dis.* 25, 1041-9.

[546] Francica, J.V.; Bigongiari, A.; Mochizuki, L.; Scapini, K.B.; Moraes, O.A.; Mostarda, C.; Caperuto, E.C.; Irgoyen, M.C.; De Angelis, K. and Rodrigues, B. (2015) Cardiac autonomic dysfunction in chronic stroke women is attenuated after submaximal exercise test, as elevated by linear and nonlinear analysis. *B.M.C. Cardiovasc. Disord.* 15, 105.

[547] Kalopita, S.; Liatis, S.; Thomakos, P.; Vlahodimitris, I.; Stathi, C.; Katsilambros, N.; Tentolouris, N. and Makrilakis, K. (2014) Relationship between autonomic nervous system function and continuous interstitial glucose measurement in patients with type 2 diabetes. *J. Diabetes Res.* 2014, 835392.

[548] Braithwaite, S.S. (2013) Glycemic variability in hospitalized patients: choosing metrics while awaiting the evidence. *Curr. Diab. Rep.* 13, 138-54.

[549] Farrokhi, F.; Chandra, P.; Smiley, D.; Pasquel, F.J.; Peng, L.; Newton, C.A. and Umpierrez, G.E. (2014) Glucose variability is an independent predictor of mortality in hospitalized patients treated with total parenteral nutrition. *Endocr. Pract.* 20, 41-5.

[550] Giordani, I.; Di Flaviani, A.; Picconi, F.; Malandrucco, I.; Yili, D.; Palazzo, P.; Altavilla, R.; Vernieri, F.; Passarelli, F.; Donno, S.; Lauro, D.; Pasqualetti, P. and Frontoni, S. (2014) Acute hyperglycemia reduces cerebrovascular reactivity: the role of glycemic variability. *J. Clin. Endocrinol. Metab.* 99, 2854-60.

[551] Jaiswal, M.; McKeon, K.; Comment, N.; Henderson, J.; Swanson, S.; Plunkett, C.; Nelson, P. and Pop-Busui, R. (2014) Association between impaired cardiovascular autonomic function and hypoglycemia in patients with type 1 diabetes. *Diabetes Care* 37, 2616-21.

[552] Prázný, M. and Soupal, J. (2014) Glycemic variability and continuous monitoring of glycemia. *Vnitr. Lek.* 60, 757-63.

[553] Hayes, M.A.; Timmins, A.C.; Yau, E.H.; Palazzo, M.; Watson, D. and Hinds, C.J. (1997) Oxygen transport patterns in patients with sepsis syndrome or septic shock: influence of treatment and relationship to outcome. *Crit. Care Med.* 25, 926-36.

[554] Niederer, D.; Vogt, L.; Gonzalez-Rivera, J.; Schmidt, K. and Banzer, W. (2015) Heart rate recovery and aerobic endurance capacity in cancer survivors: interdependence and exercise-induced improvements. *Support Care Cancer* 23, 3513-20.

[555] Torella, M.; Castells, I.; Gimenez-Perez, G.; Recasens, A.; Miquel, M.; Simó, O.; Barbeta, E. and Sampol, G. (2015) Intermittent hypoxia is an independent marker of poorer glycemic control in patients with uncontrolled type 2 diabetes. *Diabetes Metab.* 41, 312-8.

[556] Leong, W.B.; Banerjee, D.; Nolen, M.; Adab, P.; Thomas, GN. and Taheri, S. (2014) Hypoxemia and glycemic control in type 2 diabetes mellitus with extreme obesity. *J. Clin. Endocrinol. Metab.* 99, E1650-4.

[557] Rashidian, M.; Keliher, E.J.; Bilate, A.M.; Duarte, J.N.; Wojtkiewicz, G.R.; Jacobsen, J.T.; Cragnolini, J.; Swee, L.K.; Victora, G.D.; Weissleder, R. and Ploegh, H.L. (2015) Noninvasive imaging of immune responses. *Proc. Natl. Acad. Sci. USA*, 112, 6146-51.

[558] Walsh, D. and Nelson, K.A. (2002) Autonomic nervous system dysfunction in advanced cancer. *Support Care Cancer* 10, 523-8.

[559] Kortelainen, J.; Jia, X.; Seppänen, T. and Thakor, N. (2012) Increased electroencephalographic gamma activity reveals awakening from isoflurane anaesthesia in rats. *Br. J. Anaesth.* 109, 782-9.

[560] Straus, S.M.; Sturkenboom, M.C.; Bleumink, G.S.; Dieleman, J.P.; van der Lei, J.; de Graeff, P.A.; Kingma, J.H. and Stricker, B.H. (2005) Non-

cardiac QTc-prolonging drugs and the risk of sudden cardiac death. *Eur. Heart J.* 26, 2007-12.

[561] Suefke, S.; Djonlagić, H. and Kibbel, T. (2012) [Severe bacterial infection: increased mortality in elderly women with low body weight taking drugs prolonging the QTc interval]. *Med. Klin. Intensivmed. Notfmed.* 107, 275-84.

[562] Vrtovec, B.; Okrajsek, R.; Golicnik, A.; Ferjan, M.; Starc, V. and Radovancevic, B. (2005) Atorvastatin therapy increases heart rate variability, decreases QT variability, and shortens QTc interval duration in patients with advanced chronic heart failure. *J. Card. Fail.* 11, 684-90.

[563] Kim, E.; Joo, S.; Kim, J.; Ahn, J.; Kim, J.; Kimm, K. and Shin, C. (2006) Association between C-reactive protein and QTc interval in middle-aged men and women. *Eur. J. Epidemiol.* 21, 653-9.

BIOGRAPHICAL SKETCH

Thomas Kibbel, MD PhD

Affiliation:
1. University Clinic Schleswig-Holstein, Campus Luebeck, Medical Department I
2. LAFAA Laboratory for Contract Research in Clinical Pharmacology and Pharmaceutical Analytics GmbH, Bad Schwartau, Germany

Address:
D-23538 Luebeck
Ratzeburger Allee 160, Germany
Email: th.kibbel@gmx.de

Education:
Studies of Pharmacy and Medicine

Research and Professional Experience:
Clinical Pharmacy, Internal Medicine, Intensive Care Medicine, Clinical Studies and Pharmaceutical Bioanalytics

Professional Appointments:
Autonomic Nervous System, Heart Rate Variability, QT Prolongation, Sepsis, Gender

Last Publications:

1. Suefke, S.; Djonlagić, H. and Kibbel, T. Severe Sepsis and Septic Shock: Different Concepts of Analgesia and Sedation May Have Important Influences on Prognosis and Therapy Management. In: Graver, B. (ed.) Septic Shock: Risk Factors, Management and Prognosis, Chapter 2. Nova Science Publishers, Inc. New York 2015. ISBN 978-1-63463-916-3, pp. 27-60.
2. Suefke, S.; Djonlagić, H. and Kibbel, T. Severe Hyperglycemic Disarrangements: Heart Rate Variability as a Tool for Risk Estimation and Therapy Management. In: Berhardt, L.V. (ed.) Advances in Medicine and Biology. Volume 86. Chapter 3. Nova Science Publishers, Inc. New York 2015, ISBN 978-1-63483-007-2, pp. 31-66.
3. Suefke, S.; Djonlagić, H. and Kibbel, T. Analgesia and Sedation in Severe Sepsis and Septic Shock: A Comparison of Fentanyl/Midazolam vs. Sufentanil/Midazolam. In: Turner, A, and Hall, J. (eds.) Antibiotic Therapy: New Developments. Chapter 1. Nova Science Publishers, Inc. New York 2013, ISBN: 978-1-62808-170-1, pp. 1-62.
4. Kibbel, T.; Djonlagić, H. and Suefke, S. Gender Aspects in Septic Patients Receiving QTc Prolonging Drugs. In: Bennington, E.H. (ed.) Horizons in World Cardiovascular Research. Volume 5. Chapter 3. Nova Science Publishers, Inc. New York 2013, ISBN 978-1-62618-984-3, pp. 65-90.
5. Kibbel, T.; Djonlagić, H. and Suefke, S. Cardiac Impairment in Therapy with Fluoroquinolones. In: Berhardt, L.V. (ed.) Advances in Medicine and Biology. Volume 64. Chapter 5. Nova Science Publishers, Inc. New York 2013, ISBN: 978-1-62417-927-3, pp. 189-212.
6. Kibbel, T.; Djonlagić, H. and Suefke, S. Alcohol Induced Impairment of Cardiac Autonomic Nervous System and its Prognostic Relevance. In: Maars, J.V. (ed.) Alcohol Dependence and Addiction. Chapter 1. Nova Science Publishers, Inc. New York 2011, ISBN: 978-1-61324-796-9, pp. 1-30.

7.   Suefke, S.; Djonlagić, H. and Kibbel, T. Monitoring of Antidepressant Therapy by Using Heart Rate Variability. In: Cheng, D. and Liu, G. (eds.) Encyclopedia of Pharmacology Research (2 Volume Set). Vol. 1, Chapter 3. Nova Science Publishers, Inc. New York 2011, ISBN: 978-1-61470-405-8, pp. 93-115.

In: Autonomic Nervous System (ANS) ISBN: 978-1-63484-884-8
Editor: Patrick Bernard Owens © 2016 Nova Science Publishers, Inc.

Chapter 3

ENTRUSTING COMMUNICATION OF MENTAL AND PHYSICAL SATISFACTION AND STATE OF HEALTH TO THE AUTONOMIC NERVOUS SYSTEM

*Hiroaki Okawai**

Civil and Environmental Engineering, Graduate School of Engineering,
Iwate University 4-3-5 Ueda, Morioka, Iwate, Japan

ABSTRACT

Most of the time, we do not have a good level of awareness of the overall state of our own health. Nor do we necessarily want others to know about it if we know that we are in poor health. However, there currently exists neither an objective scale nor satisfactory terminology to describe an individual's general state of health, which makes it difficult to articulate. For this reason, the author studied non-verbal communication of individuals' physiological condition during periods of unconsciousness – i.e., during sleep.

In daily life we accept various services, and the suppliers thereof usually want to know to what extent customers were satisfied with the services provided. However, a range of constraints mean that we do not always provide an honest response. Moreover, customers are sometimes

* Corresponding author: hokawai@iwate-u.ac.jp, Tel/fax: +81-19-621-6318. hokw38-hiroaki5@memoad.jp

unaware of services accepted. In questionnaire responses, for example, the customer's feedback vis-à-vis services received is, for various reasons, often distorted. The same is true of cases pertaining to health and satisfaction, and problems may be caused by mental activity, i.e., consciousness. The notion of entrusting the response to a service to the autonomic nervous system during sleep has therefore been suggested and demonstrated.

It is known that both respiration and pulse during sleep are controlled by the autonomic nervous system. To investigate respiration and pulse, a pressure sensor was used. The pressure signal was conceptualized as the body motion wave (BMW). As well as enabling a broader understanding of the autonomic nervous system, this method also enabled investigation of sleeping posture and body action. The method was initially confirmed using stimuli of aroma and music, since these are known to be conducive to relaxation. The autonomic nervous system responded to the relaxation effect (satisfaction) with a decrease in respiration and pulse rates. The same method was then applied to evaluation of other services, e.g., bedding materials, both on the market and those in development, to gather data on the autonomic nervous system's responses. These materials were thus classified according to satisfaction as expressed by physical activity rather than mental activity.

On the basis of this study, more of control was studied. It was found that the respiratory and cardiovascular systems are controlled in a different manner during periods of increase and decrease. Linked to this, changes in sleeping posture occur not in a random order but, as it were, in a physiological order, that is, a trigger to increase or decrease respiration and/or pulse rate rapidly in a wide range. Subsequently, the question of why and how the rate increases and decreases periodically was investigated by studying the instantaneous pulse rate. The results indicate that the pulse rate does not remain constant, but varies, with roughly three pulse rate ranges per minute, and fluctuates significantly at both higher and lower rate ranges.

1. WHAT IS HEALTH?

1.1. Information about Health

Health is a matter of public concern. From the viewpoint of biological measurement for diseases, details of the body's pathology, along with methods for examining it, have been well studied, and various scales determined. However, measurement of everyday physical condition has not yet been studied to any significant degree, since variation in the body's condition in the range of "not abnormal" in the medical view is neither easily detectable nor easy to recognize in oneself.

The state of "not abnormal" does not mean "healthy", and for this reason, measuring variations in condition within the "not abnormal" state – i.e., unknown to the individual concerned – has become a significant theme in current research. If a slight variation in body condition in daily life can be detected it may be possible to thwart the onset of a serious illness, something of heightened importance in an aging society. Furthermore, it would enable the formulation of efficient everyday work and holiday schedules, and to implement precautions orientated toward accident prevention.

1.2. It Is Health That People Desire

In Japan, particularly in the period between 1945 and 1990, there was a need for commodities such as food, clothing, and housing. Various technologies were developed to advance sanitation, health, beauty, security, information, recreation, and so forth. Refrigerators, television sets and washing machines in particular heralded a revolution in day-to-day living. This was a period, in other words, during which material things were able to satisfy people's wishes, and food, clothing and housing thus went a long way toward creating both physical and mental satisfaction. What people were afraid of was perhaps sudden or painful death, for example due to cancer, heart disease or stroke, unavoidable by means of material goods.

However, research conducted by an insurance company in the 2000s revealed that what people feared most was dementia, or becoming bedridden – more so than death from illness or accident – suggesting that people nowadays lack in satisfaction of mind, which in turn results in a preoccupation with our health and that of our families and friends.

1.3. What Is Health?

In 1945 (revised in 1998) the World Health Organization (WHO) defined "health" as "a dynamic state of complete physical, mental, spiritual and social well-being and not merely the absence of disease or infirmity."

Given the deeper meaning attributed to health in this definition, the present study focuses on the following assertions:

1. Health does not mean that we are healthy unless we are ill.
2. The condition of being "well" means being healthy but does not cover every aspect of health.

For this reason, the focus of the present study is the issue of what health is and how is it determined. The following sections will outline a trial for this purpose by developing a method for measuring mental and physical condition, as opposed to illness, through the study of sleep and the autonomic nervous system, and as pertaining to health and satisfaction with a service.

2. USING SLEEP TO OBTAIN INFORMATION ABOUT HEALTH

2.1. Method for Obtaining Unconscious Output

Usually we do not have a good level of awareness either of our general state of health or the condition of our body. Equally, for reasons of modesty or other individual constraints, if we are aware that we are in poor health we sometimes do not want others to know. On the other hand, people who need to be particularly careful about managing their own health – athletes, drivers, control room staff etc. – need to have a thorough understanding of their own state of health. However, there is currently neither a scale nor the terminology to describe it, and there is thus no easy way of expressing an individual's overall state of health.

For this reason, the author looked to non-verbal communication through physiological behaviors during states of unconsciousness, i.e., during sleep. The measurement method can be employed at home and without the need for the involvement of medical professionals.

This new method, developed in the current study, entrusts communication of the individual's physical condition to the autonomic nervous system during sleep. The method constitutes a new, highly accurate method of measurement of the activities of the autonomic nervous system, using information such as pulse rate, respiration, and sleeping posture.

Information regarding unconscious activities can also to some extent be obtained during periods of consciousness; however, it is significantly masked during these periods by the effects of the mind, e.g., white coat hypertension.

The purity of unconscious activities during sleep, on the other hand, is much higher than in a waking state. Figure 2.1 suggests a human system that produces conscious and unconscious outputs in response to stimuli in consciousness and unconsciousness.

Broadly speaking, brain function – i.e., the human system depicted in this model – consists of the interaction between the mind function and body function. It then has conscious and unconscious outputs delineated by a diagonal dashed line. Output 1 is for language and Output 2 for motion, controlled by conscious activities, while Outputs 3 to 5 are for unconscious activities. Then, the characteristics of the human system are exposed more when some stimuli input as shown by Sc, for the conscious one, and Su for unconscious ones. This idea is based on systems engineering's notion of the flow of input – characteristics – output.

For this reason, sleep is expected to be the means by which to obtain the unconscious output of Outputs 3 and 5.

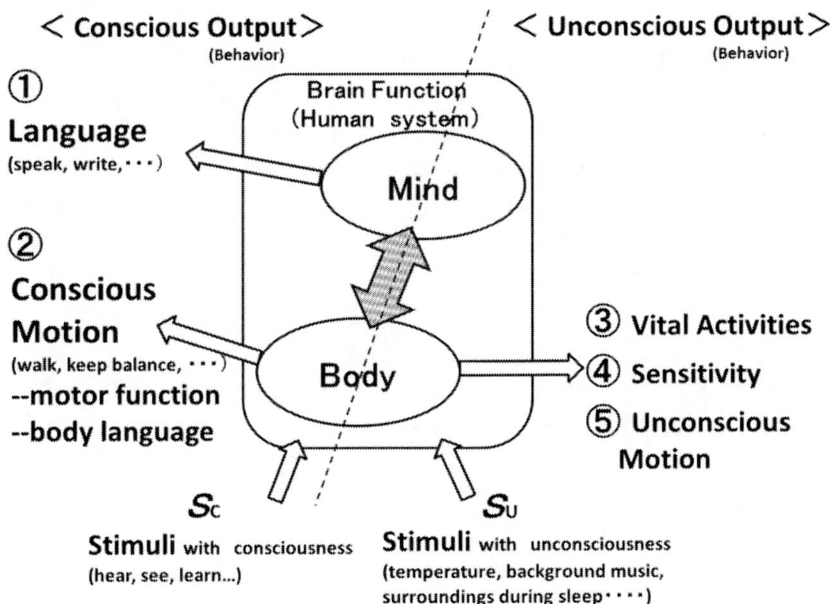

Figure 2.1. Hypothetical model of the human system revealing conscious and unconscious outputs, produced by interactions between mind and body, in response to stimuli.

2.2. Method for Obtaining Honest Information about Health

Here, it is important to understand what sleep is, from the viewpoint of conventional physiology.

Meaning 1: Sleep restores a human being, both physically and mentally – a well-established fact in physiology.

REM sleep and non-REM sleep occur alternately and rhythmically over the course of a sleeping period; hormones such as melatonin are secreted to promote good sleep, as well as growth hormones for tissue growth and restoration. In another words, good sleep enables the restoration of the body and mind and enables the human being to maintain a good overall level of health.

This physiology also means that the information given out during sleep will contain information about the condition of the body or general state of health. The author has therefore gathered sleep data for more than 600 nights for a total of more than 150 subjects over the course of ten years, so as to gain an understanding of the following:

Meaning 2: Sleep reveals information regarding the condition of the body or general state of health (the findings from the present study).

As described in the following section, with regard to the study of health along with satisfaction – i.e., results of mental and physical activities from the viewpoint of sleep – it was experimentally confirmed that mental and physical activities are closely linked. Therefore, as stated in the next section, the study of health together with satisfaction may provide a way of easily understanding health.

3. SLEEP AS A MEANS OF OBTAINING INFORMATION ABOUT SERVICE AND SATISFACTION

3.1. Introduction

Suppliers of the services we receive in our everyday lives often want feedback on customer satisfaction. However, due to a range of possible constraints, recipients of a service do not always give an honest response as to whether or not they are satisfied, and, as mentioned in section 2.1, this is also true in the case of health. Moreover, customers are sometimes not aware of the services accepted. Although questionnaire survey, for example, is often adopted, the customer's responses, for one reason or another, are often distorted, and hence neither accurate nor honest.

Therefore, the question here is whether or not it is possible for suppliers to gain a clear picture of customer satisfaction on the basis of accurate and/or honest responses to the services provided and thus improve the services on the basis of customer feedback. To resolve such problems, Okawai et al. [1][2][3][4] have suggested a method to entrust feedback to unconscious responses through signs of vital activities, for example, rates of respiration and pulse, reflecting the activities of the autonomic nervous system during sleep, paying attention to non-verbal communication through physiological behavior in states of unconsciousness.

3.2. Method for Obtaining Data of Unconscious Responses

(1) Model of the Human System from the Input/Output Viewpoint

Generally speaking, a system is a mechanism for producing an output, i.e., a response to stimuli modulated by the characteristics of that system. This idea has been applied to the human system [1] [2] [3] [4]. A human is an elaborate system, with two functions – mental and physical activities – as shown in a schematic function model in Figure 3.1 with reference to Figure 2.1. Service, to a human, is a stimulus as described above. Therefore, the human receives a stimulus, i.e., input of service, intentionally or unintentionally, through the individual's own various biological sensors, bringing one or both of the abovementioned functions into action in the output of a response. For the output, the figure suggests a mechanism of inducing a conscious response and an unconscious response to an input of a service.

In Figure 3.1, article, information, energy, and labor are listed as examples of input. Listening, reading, watching, buying, and receiving something in a conscious state are examples of input stimuli; unconscious (i.e., unintentional) stimuli are also inputs.

Output through language, such as talking or writing, and/or conscious motion, is a conscious response, while motions due to motor function, such as walking, are conscious motion controlled by mental activity. On the other hand, variation in physical condition is an unconscious response expressed through vital activity, sensitivity, and unconscious motion.

Here, the flow to conscious response is as follows. A biological signal, produced due to sensing stimuli at channel 1 (circled 1), flows into channels 2 and 3 to activate mental activity and physical activity, respectively. These mental and physical activities then interact through channel 4. Mental activity, such as satisfaction or emotion, probably enhances physical activity. Good physical activity will also enhance mental activity.

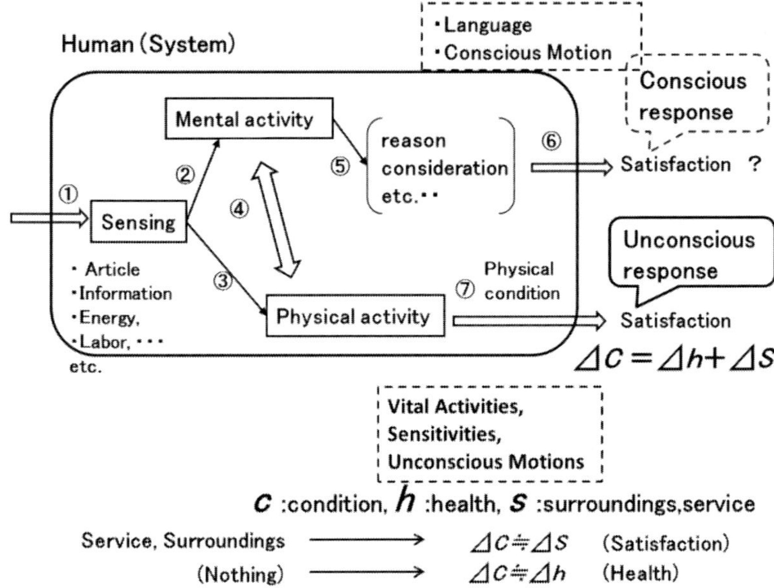

Figure 3.1. Hypothetical function model of a human system, revealing flow of a service from sensing to response.

Mental activity will thus respond to a service via a conscious response through channels 5 and 6. However, it may give a false indication of satisfaction, since a signal of mental activity may be distorted for a number of reasons as shown in the bracket between channels 5 and 6. Thus, the response may not always be accurate. In addition, mental activity does not always have a clear idea of satisfaction or otherwise. Also, for stimuli such as lower variations of temperature or background music during the unconscious state, a signal does not pass through channel 2.

On the contrary, there are two lines in the physical activity as a physical condition to express an unconscious response. One, channel 3, is direct, and the other, channel 4, via a mental activity. The signals from these two channels are combined and then sent by channel 7 for output. This output, an unconscious response – vital activities, sensitivities, unconscious movements etc. – should be an honest answer, having not been distorted for any of the reasons mentioned above.

Physical condition generating unconscious response as shown in Figure 3.1 was determined by a factor of condition c. This factor c was simply determined here by $c = hs$, where h is a factor of health and s is a factor of surroundings or service. For the lowest amount of variation, it can be simply expressed as

$$C + \mathrm{d}c = (h + \mathrm{d}h)(s + \mathrm{d}s) = (1 + \mathrm{d}h)(1 + \mathrm{d}s), \ (\mathrm{d: delta})$$
$$\mathrm{d}c = \mathrm{d}h + \mathrm{d}s.$$

As some variation of surroundings or service, $\mathrm{d}s$, is input under a state of health maintained, i.e., $\mathrm{d}h = 0$, the output will mainly occur as $\mathrm{d}c = \mathrm{d}s$. If c varied with no sensitive input, the fraction of health condition, $\mathrm{d}h$, must have varied.

(2) Classification of the Human System Model

Services as shown by channel 1 in Figure 3.1 can be roughly classified into two types as shown in Figure 3.2 [2]. The one is accepted both mentally and physically by Type-I having channels 2 and 3 from the beginning, such as articles of food, energy for getting warm or cool, etc. The other is done mentally at first by Type-II not having channel 3, for example information such as news, pictures, music, etc.

Everyday life comprises two states – waking and sleeping – as shown in Figure 3.2. In the waking state, mental activities produced in the cerebrum will generate a conscious response. The output from the mental activity is honest at channel 5; however, it is often distorted at channel 6 prior to expression as a conscious response. Although physical activity occurs via a signal at channels 4 and/or 3, an honest answer comes out as an unconscious response, though the conscious response appears superior to the unconscious response. The unconscious response can be accumulated physiologically as a physical condition, so as to be detected in the sleeping state.

In the next stage of this idea, in the sleeping state, because mental activity is at rest, the conscious response is masked. In other words, the output over several hours of sleep is free from reason, consideration etc. As a result, in the unconscious state, physical activity may be analysed with a high degree of accuracy. Vital signs such as pulse, respiration, and other unconscious responses are controlled by the activities of autonomic nervous system, superior to the activities of the other nervous systems, that is, somatic nervous systems.

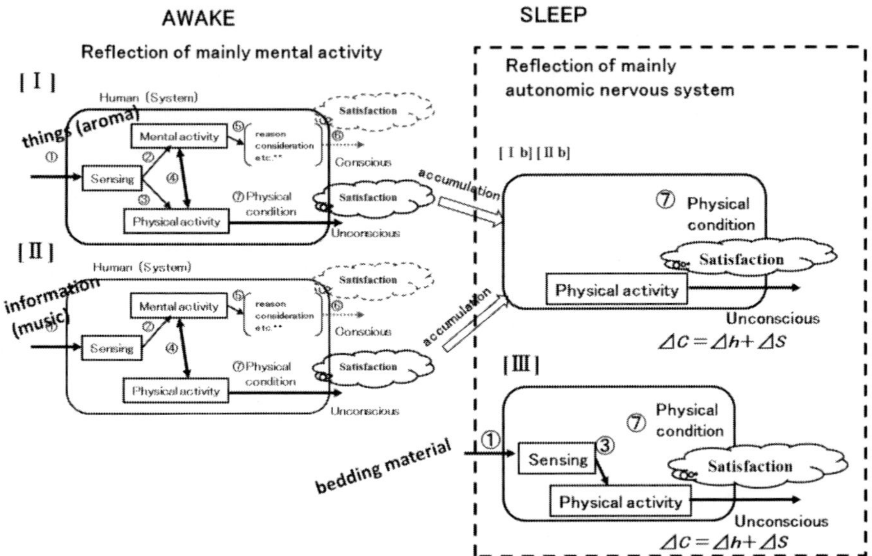

Figure 3.2. Hypothetical model revealing three types of service flows. Type-I, Type-II, and Type-III.

There is a further type of unconscious input to the human system during sleep as shown by Type-III, having neither channels 2 nor 4. The mind thus does not play a role, and the vital activities therefore express unconscious responses free from reason and other conscious motives.

In the sleep state, anxiety or poor health conditions are mitigated to some extent due to the activity of hormones; however, it seems that satisfaction accumulated physiologically can make the activity of hormones effective over the course of a sleeping period.

4. METHOD FOR MEASURING SATISFACTION OR BODY CONDITION THROUGH ACTIVITIES OF THE AUTONOMIC NERVOUS SYSTEM

4.1. Instrumentation

It is understood that both respiration and pulse during sleep are controlled by the autonomic nervous system and that their rates become lower than in the waking state: [2].

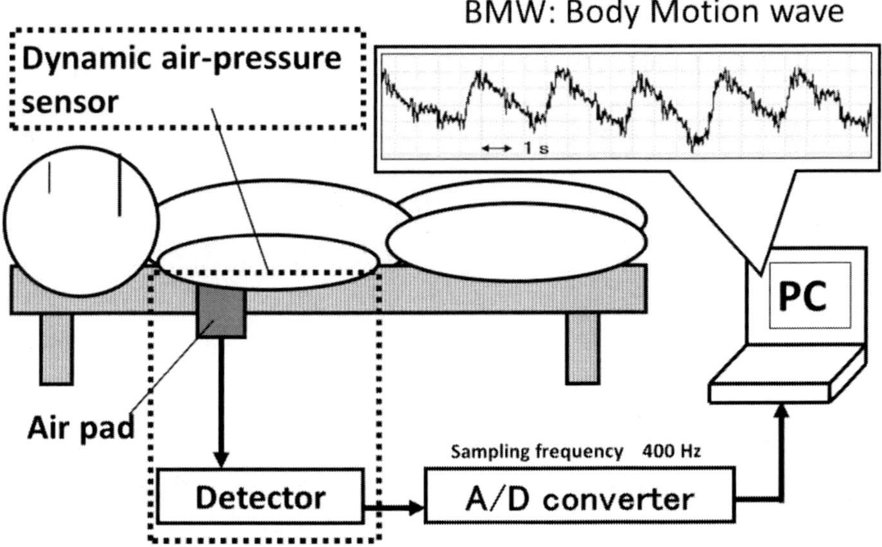

Figure 4.1. Measurement system to detect body motion wave (BMW).

In order to investigate further, a measurement system with which to detect vital activities during natural sleep has been developed [2], as shown in Figure 4.1. Natural sleep here means that a subject spends a normal day in a waking state and sleeps with no restriction, such as drugs, sensors, etc.

A pressure sensor known as a "dynamic air pressure sensor" (M. I. Labo) was adopted so as to construct a non-restraint measurement system. In principle, it was only placed on a bed in order to detect dynamic air pressure arising between the sensor and a subject's body while lying on the bed. The pressure variation detected with the sensor was converted to electric signals, the "body motion wave" (see later), sampled at the rate of 400 Hz, 16 bit, and stored in a personal computer. The signal was processed with Chart v4.2.2 (AD Instrument) and programmable software VEE Pro 6.0 (Agilent Technologies).

It is understood that vital activities (respiration, pulse etc.) occur independently, as unconscious responses free from mediation by the rational mind. The reproducibility of this system has already been confirmed [1] [2] [3] [4] as shown in section 4.3.

4.2. Body Motion Wave

As reported by Okawai et al. [1] [2] [3] [4], in a subject's body during sleep certain continuous motions are generated resulting in respiration and pulse, hence motions can be detected as a pressure wave, named "body motion wave (BMW)". This wave can be filtered out into "respiration-origin BMW (R-BMW)" and "pulse-origin BMW (P-BMW)" as shown in Figure 4.2 (a). In addition, during sleep, certain frequent extra motions are generated, resulting in unconscious actions. These can be detected as pressure waves also.

For these extra waves, two broad types of wave appear as shown in Figure 4.2(b). One was named Tremble-origin BMW (T-BMW), with a small magnitude and short duration due to a slight action of a part of the body. The other was named Action-origin BMW (A-BMW) having a large magnitude and wide duration of wave. The accuracy of this method for detecting rates of respiration and pulse has already been confirmed through comparison with data taken from a thermistor and an electrocardiogram: [5].

Thus, the present method, adopting a non-adhesive, dynamic air pressure sensor, has the following merits: (i) it can be utilized easily in everyday life because it requires no involvement by medical professionals; (ii) it obtains data throughout an entire period in bed, even if a subject, say, goes to the bathroom during the night; (iii) it collects data of pulse, respiration and movement simultaneously; and (iv) it therefore secures a subject's privacy, since neither a video camera nor microphone are used.

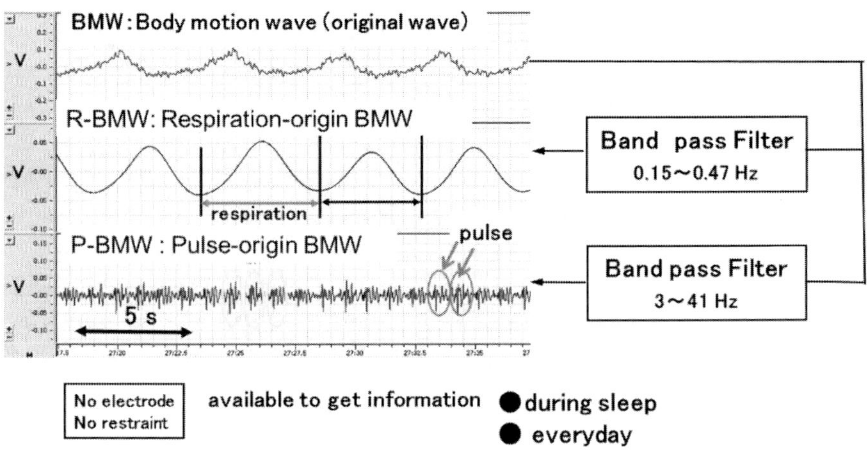

(a)

Figure 4.2. (Continued).

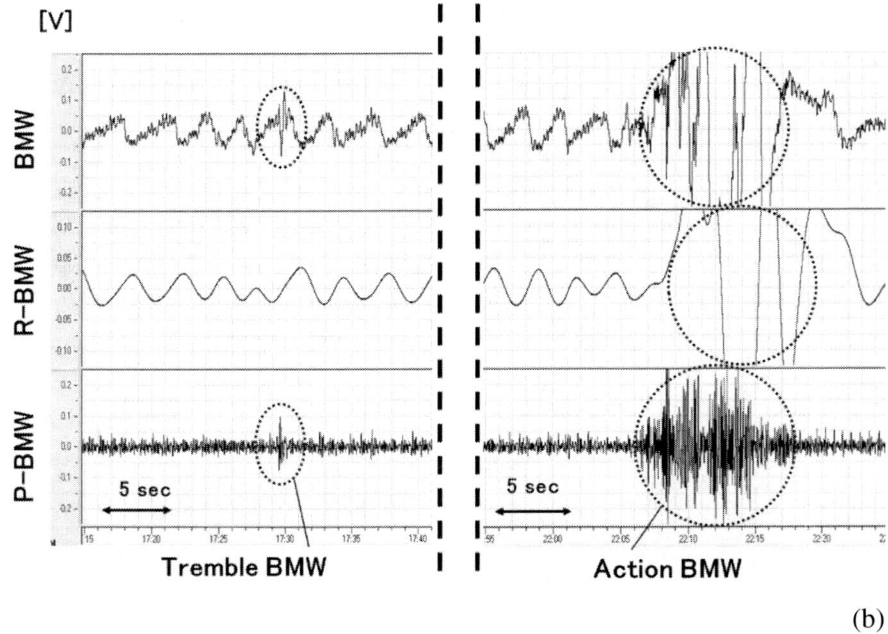

(b)

Figure 4.2. Body motion wave having components of respiration-origin BMW (R-BMW) and pulse-origin BMW (P-BMW).
(a) Body motion wave (BMW) can be filtered into components of respiration-origin and pulse-origin BMWs: R-BMW and P-BMW.
(b) Tremble BMW and Action BMW: T-BMW shows small magnitude and relatively short duration, while A-BMW shows large magnitude and longer duration.

4.3. Demonstration of Validity of BMW Method by Known Stimuli

(1) Reproducibility and Development of Accuracy in the Present Method

The sleep experiment was carried out in a unique laboratory known as the "Healthcare Experiment House" on the Iwate University campus, which replicates to the greatest extent possible the subject's normal everyday life and routines. To establish the validity of the methodology, experimental data were taken for two consecutive week nights for a subject under the following conditions: a) almost same schedule in awaking state, and b) the same environment during sleep. Thus, a result was obtained as shown in Figure 4.3. The results were as follows:

(i) The transition of the rates for both respiration and pulse showed approximately the same patterns between upper and lower figures, respectively. The respiration rate was approximately 16-18 before 3.5 h and a little higher after 3.5 h, while the pulse rate was approximately 50-60 in both the upper and lower figures.

(ii) The transition pattern showed periodicity increasing and decreasing over 60-120 minute periods depending on the individual involved.

(iii) In the case of poor physical condition due to several days' lack of sleep prior to the experiment, not shown here, a different pattern was found for the same subject.

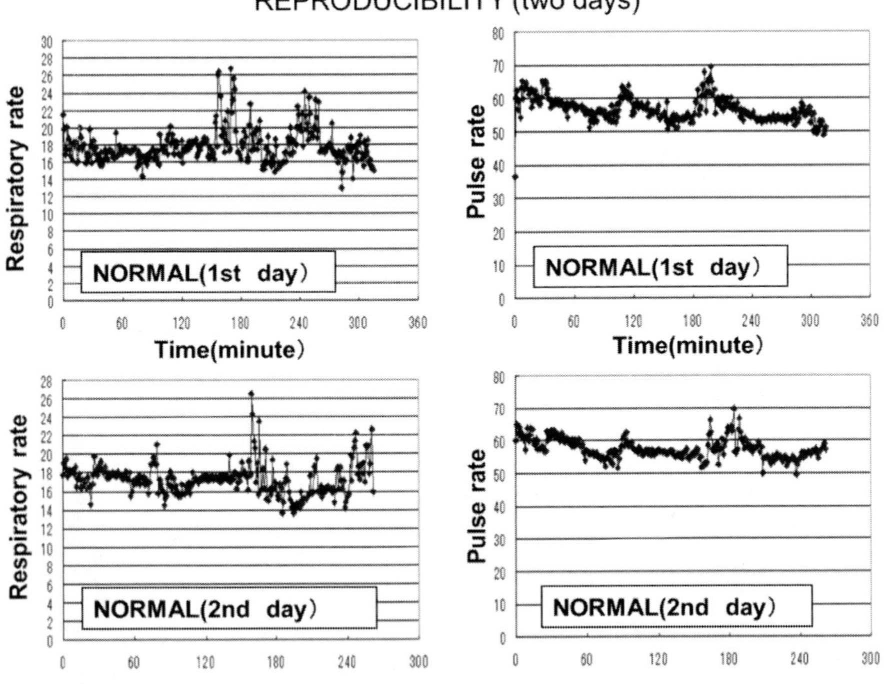

Figure 4.3. Example of rate transitions of respiration and pulse for two consecutive nights to demonstrate the reproducibility of both methodology and physiology for a normal subject. "Normal" in the figure means that a subject slept under his/her usual sleep conditions.

These findings demonstrate reproducibility in terms of both methodology and physiology for a normal subject. The study has collected data from 250+ 'normal' subjects in their 20s, and several tens of elderly subjects. However, some subjects showed different patterns of transition between the first and second nights, perhaps due to sensitivity to a change of sleeping environment. Though this difference is a kind of response to a stimuli (a change of place), data with significant difference were excluded because they were not appropriate for the purposes of this experiment, giving stimuli for the third and fourth days.

(2) Experiments for Samples for Known Stimuli

The set of experiments performed on a single subject were carried out over the course of four consecutive weekdays. The data for the first and second days as normal days were checked from the viewpoint of physiological reproducibility, and these data were used as control, as outlined in the previous section. The data at the third and fourth days, i.e., the days where stimuli were introduced, were compared with the control data. Weeks or weekends containing a national holiday or event day were excluded because of the mental or physical variations this might engender. Any subject in an unusual condition as a result of some kind of mental or physical situation was excluded.

Three types of stimuli – (a) aroma, (b) healing music, and (c) moss – were adopted for the service of healing and relaxing. The reasons for the adoption of these are as follows: it is well-established internationally that aroma and healing music have a relaxation effect. Moss has been used in temples in Japan since the Eighth Century and is recognized by Buddhists for its potential utility in achieving a state of mental detachment.

(i) For aroma, subjects who did not use aroma in their daily lives were selected. An aromatic oil that each subject liked was chosen from more than 20 different types of oil and diffused in the room approximately 1-2 h (hours) prior to the subject going to bed. The aroma remained for approximately 2-3 h after going bed. Aromatic oil is a material accepted by the sense of smell and which simultaneously relaxes the mind of the subject. Since the subject selected their oil by smell before the experiment, it also produced mental stimulation from or prior to the beginning of diffusion. Therefore, this applies to Type-I in Figure 3.2.

(ii) For healing music, subjects who did not listen to healing music in their daily lives were selected. A type of music that the subject liked was chosen from more than 30 kinds and played in the room for approximately 30 min (minutes) to 1 h between 2 h and 0.5 h before going to bed. Music is not material, but a kind of information initially accepted by the sense of hearing. Therefore, this applies to Type-II in Figure 3.2.

(iii) Moss was adopted and set in a bedding room in the experiment house for the third and fourth days. However, while the subject was aware of the presence of moss in the room they did not know why it was there, unlike the aroma and music, the aims of which were easy to understand. None of the subjects reported relaxation comparable to that induced by aroma in the waking state. Moss does not have smell, sound, or taste; therefore, the author believes that it emits something which is not perceptible via the senses. This therefore corresponds to Type-II, channel 3 in Figure 3.2 rather than channel 2.

(3) Experimental Findings for Autonomic Nervous Systems from the Viewpoint of Service

In this section, the data obtained for the items (i)-(iii) shown above are discussed. Regarding the first item, *aroma* stimuli, example transitions for a subject of pulse rate in the upper and of respiratory rate in the lower over the course of one night are shown in Figure 4.4. The left two are for the normal (control), i.e., with no particular stimulus for the first and second nights, and the right two for aroma. The results displayed in Figure 4.4 (a) show that pulse rate decreased, in particular in the first hour, while respiration rate did not decrease. Dashed lines at 60 and 70 in pulse rate traces indicate a marker to compare levels. Vertical bars reaching to zero like pillars show body actions, deleted period by minute to minute to avoid miscount of rates of pulse and respiration and to provide further information regarding sleep state. This information will be discussed in section 5.3. Figure 4.4(b) shows another example for aroma. This indicates that pulse rate decreased and that respiration remained almost the same. Thus, aroma stimuli led to a decrease in pulse rate, but produced no change in respiration rate in 3 out of 3 subjects.

Regarding the second item, *music* stimuli, as shown in Figure 4.5(a) pulse rate decreased considerably by approximately 10 Bpm, while respiration rate did not vary to such a significant degree. Another example, Figure 4.5 (b) shows indicates a decrease in both rates. The arrows n_1 to n_3 and m_1 to m_3 in Figure 4.5 (a) will be discussed in section 6. Thus, music made pulse rate decrease and made respiration rate decrease for some subjects and remained constant for others.

As regards the third item, *moss,* as shown in Figure 4.6, pulse rate decreased for 6 of 8 subjects, while respiration rate remained constant for all subjects.

These results clearly show that, for the stimuli of aroma or healing music, the rates of pulse and respiration, particularly the former, during sleep decreased. Given that aroma and healing music are an internationally recognized relaxation method, the physiological detection method using BMW in the present study fundamentally supports the understanding that pulse and respiration rates decrease through relaxation [4] [5].

However, the discrepancy between the effect on respiration rate exerted by aroma and music respectively clearly indicates that, although both bring about relaxation, aroma and music influence mind and body through different mechanisms. There may be a correlation between Type-I and Type-II as shown in 3.2. Another one, moss, potentially has the same effect as aroma.

It is clear, therefore, that the satisfaction a subject felt through mental and physical activities in a waking state due to a stimulus from aroma or music for relaxation was accumulated in the body physiologically. Thus, physical data were successfully detected through the BMW method during sleep, i.e., in the condition in which the activities of parasympathetic nerves became relatively dominant compared to during normal days.

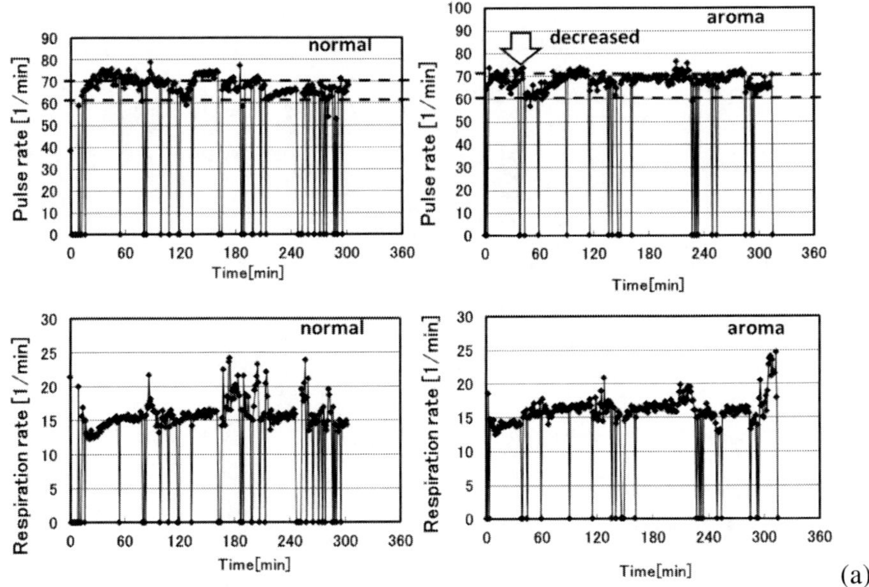

Figure 4.4. (Continued).

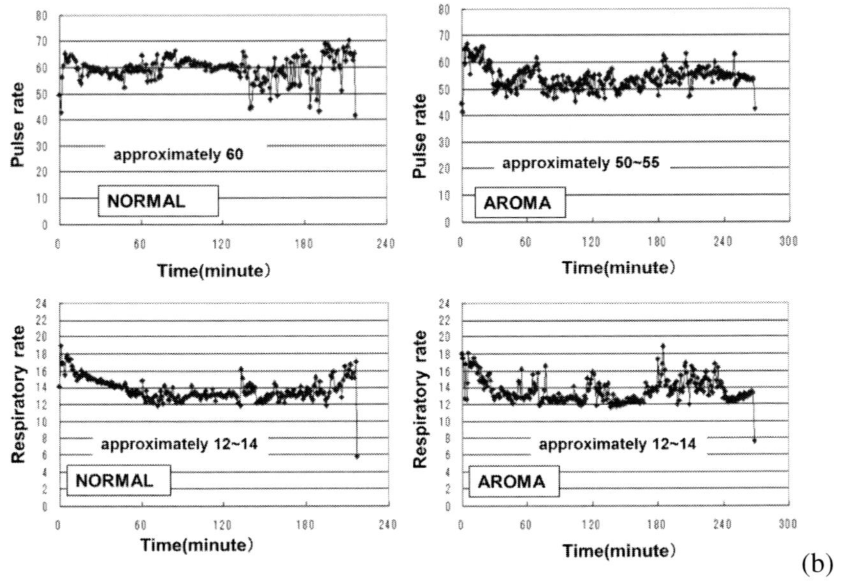

Figure 4.4. (a) (b) Rates of pulse, upper, and respiration, lower, during sleep over the course of a night. The left-hand graph shows results for "normal", i.e., with no particular service (stimulus), the right for "aroma" stimulus as a service.

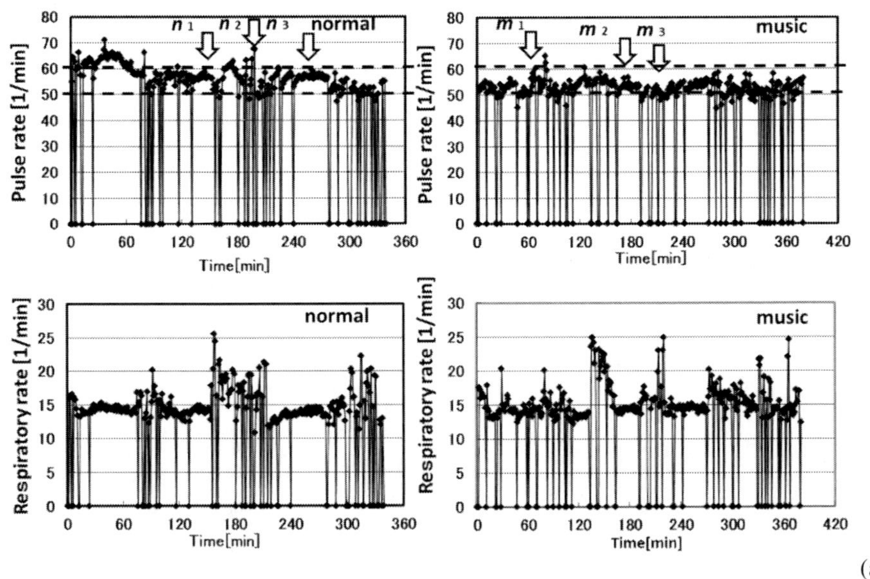

Figure 4.5. (Continued).

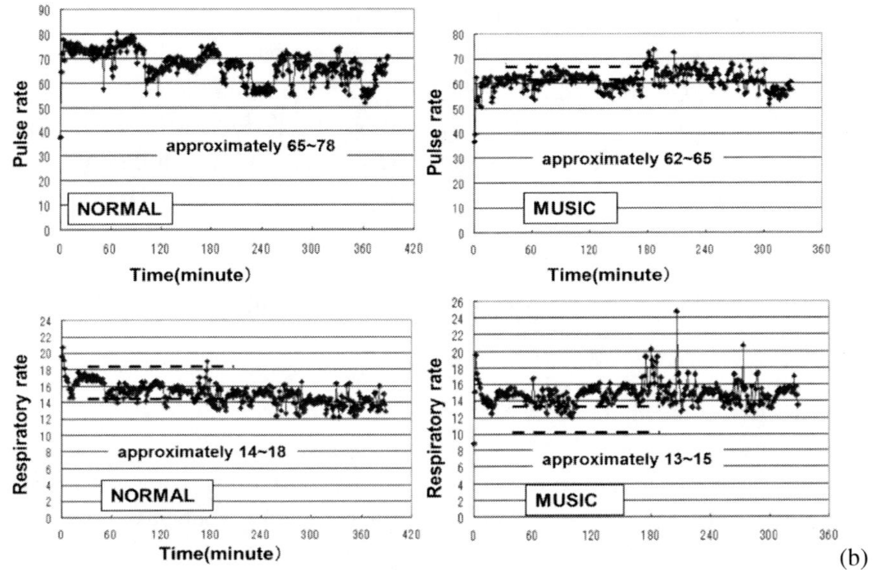

Figure 4.5. (a) (b) Rates of pulse, upper, and respiration, lower, during sleep over the course of a night. The left shows results for "normal", i.e., with no particular service (stimulus), the right for "music" stimulus as a service.

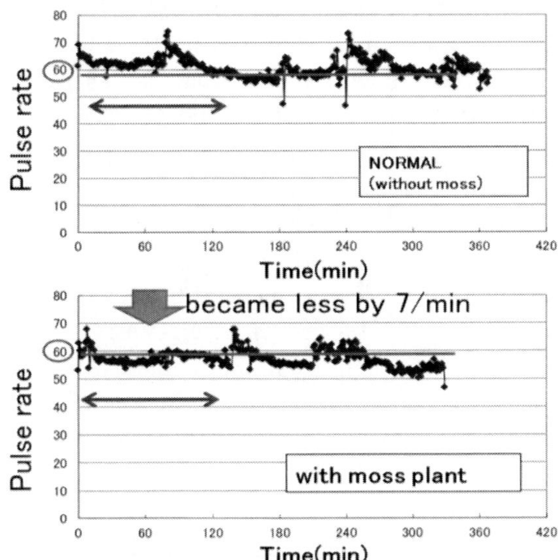

Figure 4.6. Pulse rate during sleep over the course of a night. The top graph shows results for "normal", i.e., with no particular service (stimulus), the bottom for "moss" stimulus as a service.

It is also considered that satisfaction was accumulated in mind as well as in body; however, accumulated data in the mind is masked during sleep. Thus, the method of BMW was demonstrated.

One further idea regarding Type-III in Figure 3.2, for a different process of input of stimuli/service to output of response, will be outlined in the following section.

4.4. Application of the Method to Evaluation of Bedding Materials

It is likely that all bedding materials on the market have hitherto been assessed during the waking state, i.e., during consciousness, and thus according to conscious responses to hardness, friction, color, television commercials, price, etc. It is therefore worth evaluating such materials from the viewpoint of the autonomic nervous system for the service of healing, relaxing, or improving circumstances. For this reason, a number of commercially available bedding materials were checked using the BMW method. The author also developed certain new materials.

Though a subject was, in a waking state, aware only of the name of the material to be checked and, for example, information such as low repulsion for a low repulsion mattress, this information in itself would not give a subject satisfaction or relaxation. Therefore, data obtained did not include mental activities, but rather derived only from physical sensation and physical activity. Thus, it applies to Type-III in Figure 3.2.

1. Bedding materials on the market
    Reference material was of cotton 50%, polyester 50%.
    (i) Feather (product by company A), 13 subjects.
         Pulse rate decreased for 9, remained constant for 1, and increased for 3, while respiration rate remained unchanged. Power of frequency component range of respiration, less than approx. 3Hz, over that of pulse range, i.e., heartbeat range of 4-10Hz was considerably larger.
    (ii) Low repulsion mattress (product by company B), 3 subjects.
         Pulse rate decreased for all three subjects; however, respiration rate did not vary. It was found to be hard to change sleeping posture. Respiration rate did not vary.
2. Bedding materials currently in development

(iii) Resin-1: 6 subjects.
  Pulse rate decreased for 5 subjects and did not vary for 2 subjects.
  Respiration rate did not vary.
(iv) Resin-2: 7 subjects.
  Pulse rate decrease for one subject and did not vary for 6 subjects.
  Respiration rate did not vary.
(v) Carbon: [6]

Carbon A and carbon B were tested. The experiment was carried out for four consecutive weekdays, the first two normal days, the second two the trials. Holidays were excluded due to the mental or physical variations they might induce. For this reason, the entire experiment was carried out for material A and material B over four days. Comparison of carbon and normal material was done on a separate day.

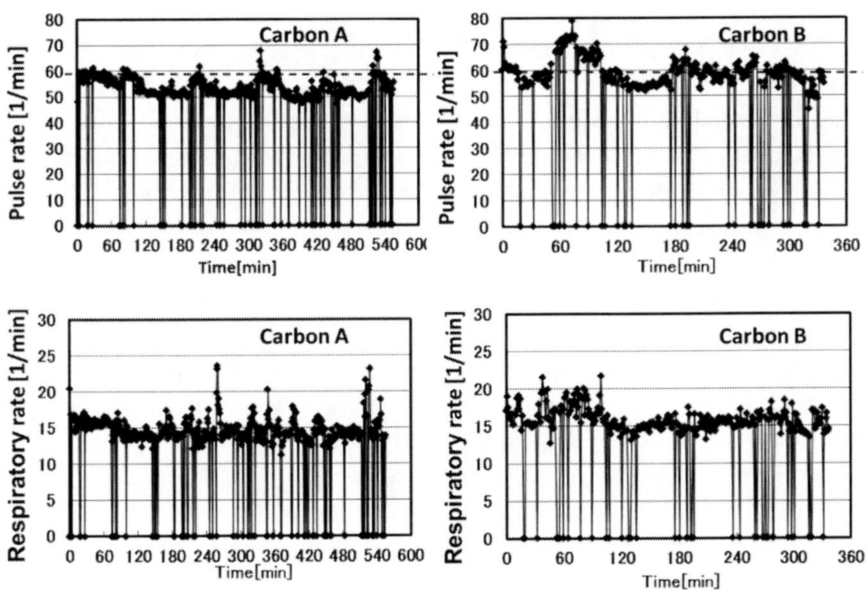

Figure 4.7. Rates of pulse for carbon A and carbon B values on workdays.

Figure 4.7 shows that pulse rate for carbon A was lower (approximately 50-60) than that of carbon B (55-70). Respiration rate for carbon A showed a value lower than around 15, while that for carbon B showed a value higher than 15. This tendency was demonstrated in three of four subjects in the 21-25 age group. Thus, it is clear that subjects expressed satisfaction definitively through their unconscious response, without mediation by mental activity processes shown by type III in Figure 3.2. The carbon material neither gave off an aroma nor had different hardness. i.e., the subject was mentally not aware of the carbon.

For this reason, although the exact bodily mechanism by which all three types of services can relax a human subject as shown in Figure 3.2 is still unknown, the usefulness or accuracy of the BMW method was demonstrated.

5. CONTROL OF RATES OF RESPIRATION AND PULSE, AND OF CHANGE IN SLEEPING POSTURE

5.1. Introduction

It is well known that respiration is performed by motions of the diaphragm and related muscles (the respiratory system), and pulse, i.e., heartbeat, by heart muscles (the cardiovascular system), related to the autonomic nervous system. However, the respiratory system is also linked to the musculoskeletal system, which is related to the cerebrum. These two activities − of the autonomic nervous system through involuntary muscles and of the cerebrum through voluntary muscles − are (I) unconscious activity and (II) conscious activity, respectively.

During sleep then, i.e., in the state of relaxation, both respiration and pulse are controlled by the autonomic nervous system, and the rates of the two decrease [7] [8]. However, phenomena that occur during sleep are not yet fully understood; it has not been established, for example, whether both respiration and pulse are controlled in the same way. If not, we are interested in what the differences are, and why and how they manifest.

There is also so far no detailed understanding of why and how sleeping posture changes. Change of sleeping posture requires certain striated muscles to work under the unconscious state; however, these muscles work voluntarily during the waking state, with the exception of respiration and pulse related activity.

In this respect, it has been reported that the autonomic nervous system works on the cardiovascular and respiratory systems in a different way [9][10], as will be described further in the following section. We studied more detailed phenomena by means of the body motion wave (BMW) so as to address some of these questions.

5.2. Slope and Periodicity in the Rate Transitions of Respiration and Pulse

Experiments were carried out with more than 70 subjects, ranging in age from 20 to 80 years. A subject usually stayed at Healthcare Experimental House in Iwate University for four consecutive nights. On the first and second days, physical reproducibility was checked with the subjects receiving no particular stimuli, and on the third and fourth days an experimental condition was changed with aim of finding a theme.

Thus, 70 nights' data obtained from 20 healthy subjects in their 20s were analyzed in detail. All of the subjects subscribed to our privacy policy. During these experiment days, subjects had a full, normal day, went to bed as usual, and awoke naturally.

Examples of the rate transitions of respiration and pulse are shown in Figure 5.1 and Figure 5.2, respectively. In Figure 5.1, a considerable number of small deletions traced like pillars getting to zero show count error due to T-BMW or A-BMW as described in Figure 4.4(a). Such deletions were interpolated to be viewed later from a different viewpoint.

The results demonstrated as follows:

(i) Transition patterns were roughly classified into three:
    a. The rate moved downward with time as shown in the upper traces of Figure 5.1 and Figure 5.2,
    b. it remained constant as shown in the lower traces, respectively, and
    c. it moved a little bit upward though not shown here.
    The data were summarized to be, in percentage, roughly 20, 70, 10 for the respiration rate and 60, 30, 10 for the pulse rate, up to now, as shown in Table 5.1. The dominant pattern was constant for respiration and downward for pulse. Thus, the transition patterns between respiration and pulse were not always same even in one subject.

(ii) Periodicity was recognized, and it indicated a difference between respiration and pulse.

It was initially confirmed that the transitions had periodicity by the increase and decrease of each rate traced over one-minute periods, i.e., minute respiration rate and minute pulse rate. It is noted that the period did not remain constant, but varied throughout a night, both for respiration and pulse, even for a subject with the range approximately 30-130 per minute, as shown for example in Figure 5.2 and Figure 5.3.

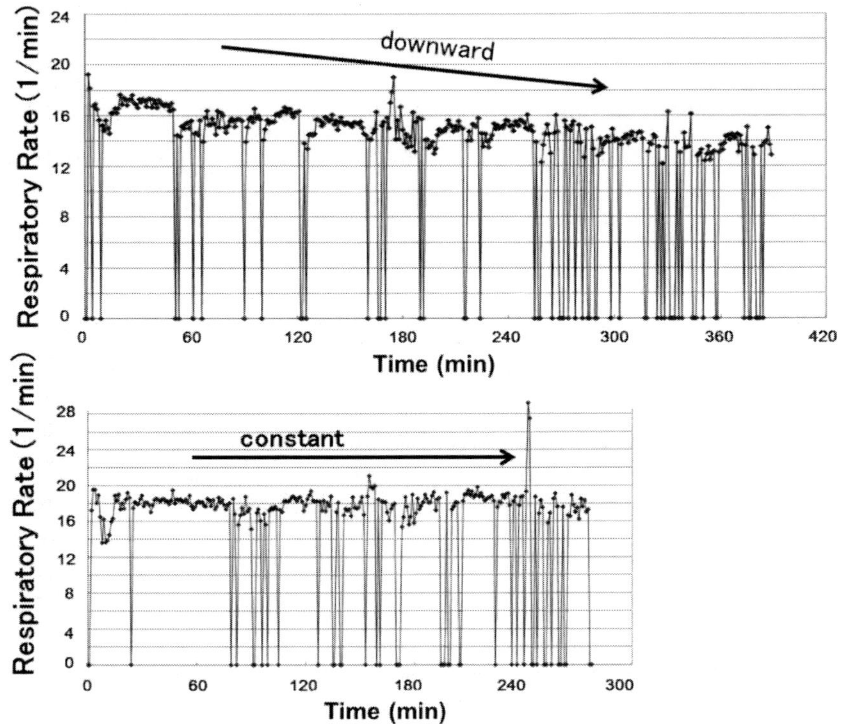

Figure 5.1. Transitions of respiration rate for two subjects.

Table 5.1. Transition patterns of two rates of respiration and pulse classified

Transition pattern	Respiration (%)	Pulse (%)
downward	20	60
Constant	70	30
Upward	10	10

As shown in Figure 5.3 for one subject, periods between transitions of the rates of respiration and pulse did not always agree with each other. This figure also shows, in contrast to the roughly constant pattern for respiration, the downward pattern for pulse mentioned in Table 1.

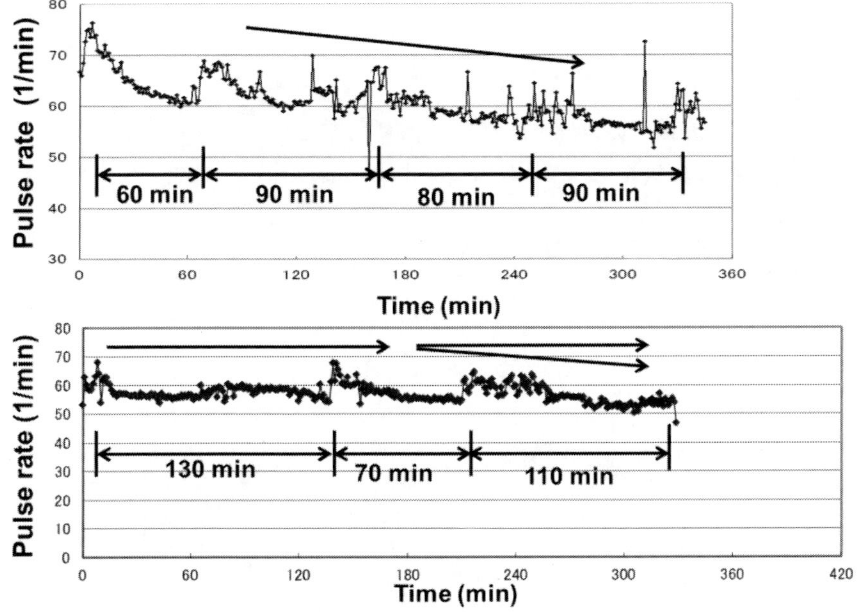

Figure 5.2. Transitions of pulse rate for two subjects.

For periodicity, in traditional sleep research using polysomnography, adopting mainly electric signals such as Electroencephalogram, sleep depth has been well explained. It has been described that the depth of sleep varies periodically in approximately 80 to 100, and typically 90 minute under the control of autonomic nervous system [9][10].

In the present study, by way of BMW due to dynamics of air pressure, the periodicity was confirmed. Therefore, it is clear that the autonomic nervous system is what makes muscles related to respiration and pulse work. However, as shown in Figure 5.3, the periods in two rate transitions were not same, and pulse here was somewhat clearer. So far it can be considered that the autonomic nervous system controls priority to pulse rate compared with respiratory rate from the viewpoint of rate. Stroke volume or cardiac output in the heart and tidal volume in the lung are beyond the scope of this study. In any case, it was found that the autonomic nervous system controls respiration and pulse in a different way. Moreover, as the respiratory system is controlled both consciously and unconsciously, the mechanism whereby it is controlled being different to that of the cardiovascular system makes it impossible for the autonomic nervous system to control the two systems in same manner.

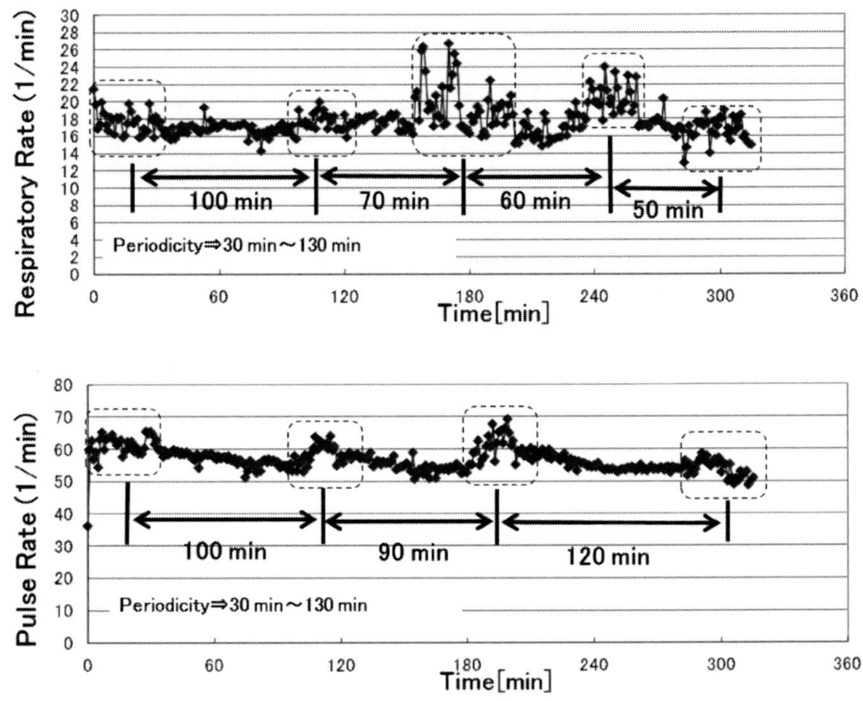

Figure 5.3. Transitions of rates of respiration and pulse for one subject to demonstrate different periodicity.

5.3. Role of Body Actions and Change of Sleeping Posture

(1) Body Actions Illustrated in the Present Study

As shown in Figure 5.1, body actions were illustrated by a significant number of pillars, vertical bars reaching to zero, deletions including mere action and change of sleeping posture, showing that there occurred T-BMW and A-BMW as mentioned in Figure 4.2(b). Therefore, though there are usually more than 60 pillars, the actual number of T-BMW and A-BMW was more than that of the pillars, reaching as high as several hundred over the course of a night.

Transition of the rate of actual number of T-BMW and A-BMW over the course of a night was, on average, in the range of approximately once or twice per minute [3] as shown, for example, in the upper trace in Figure 5.4. The time duration of action per minute ranged from approximately 5 s to 30 s, as shown in the lower trace. The transition showed that actions did not occur so much between 50 and 160 minute and occurred rather frequently after 160 minute.

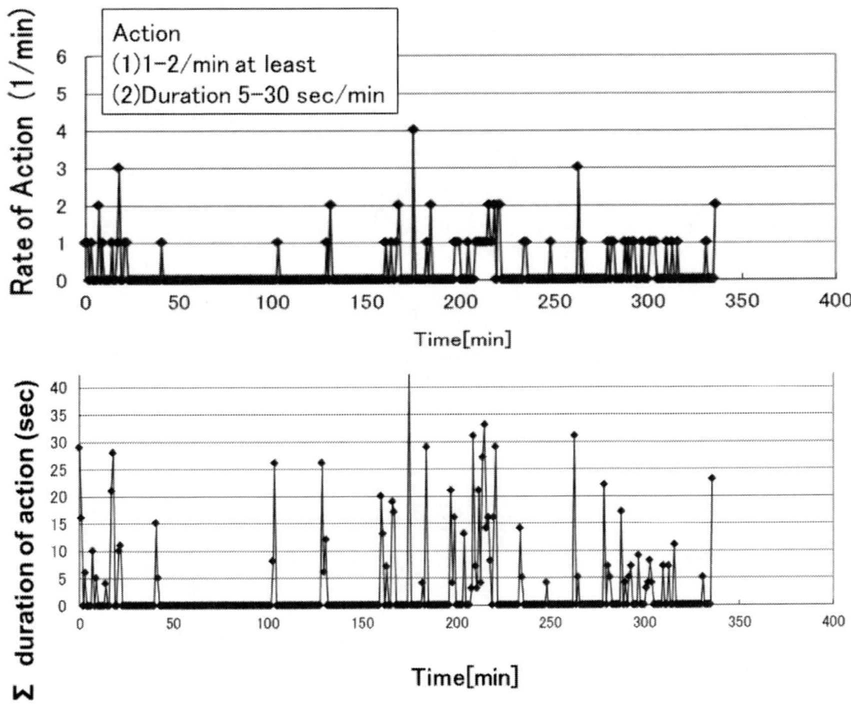

Figure 5.4. Transition of action for one night from the viewpoint of rate and duration, per one minute.

(2) Change of Sleeping Posture

The change of sleeping posture in the actions described above was detected through A-BMW and confirmed using a commercially-available pressure sensor, as shown in Figure 5.5. The A-BMW numerical data showed that all healthy subjects in their 20s changed their sleeping postures at least once per hour throughout the course of a night: to be more specific, more than four times per hour for 20% of the subjects, two or three times for 70% and once for 10%. It is particularly noteworthy that there was not a single subject who did not change his/her posture in the course of a night's sleep [9].

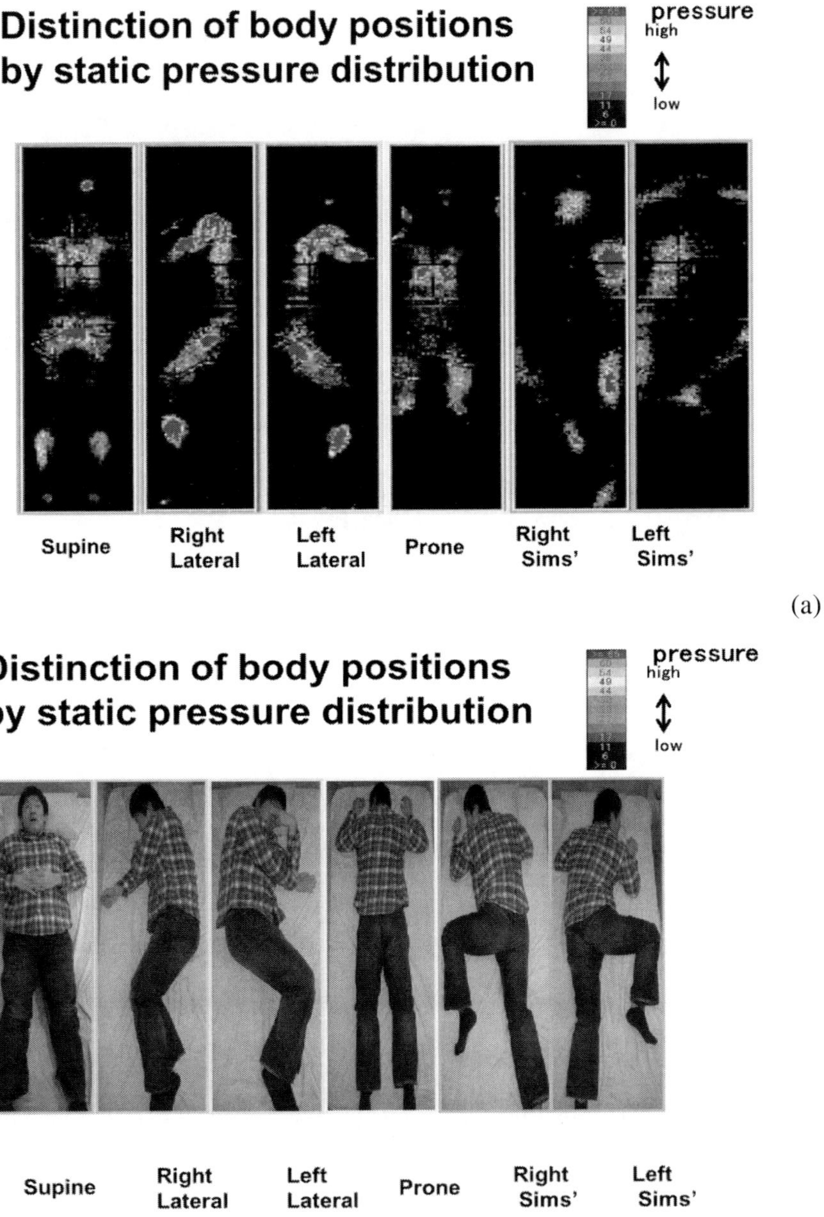

Figure 5.5. (a) Six patterns of sleeping posture (body position) detected by a commercially available pressure sensor array instrument and (b) corresponding photos.

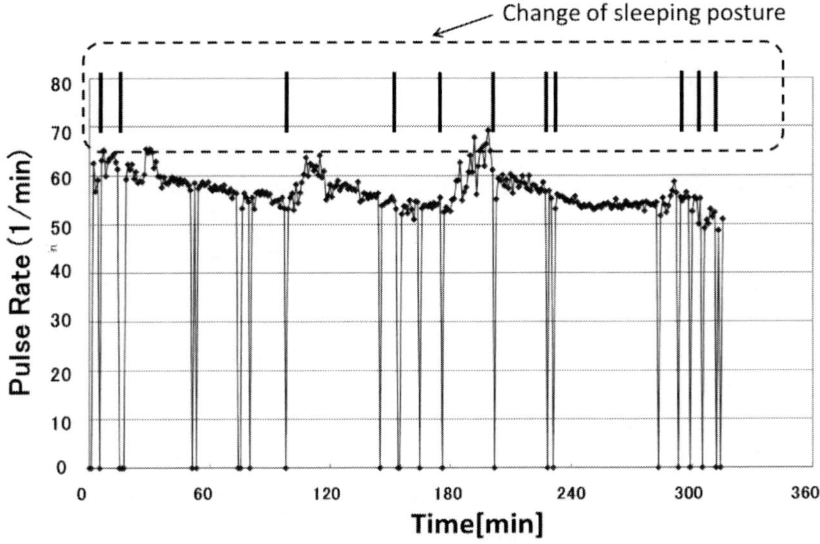

Figure 5.6. Transition of all actions described by pillars, as mentioned in Figure 5.1, along the pulse rate transition as in Figure 5.3, with the transition of change in sleeping posture added by vertical thick lines above the pulse rate.

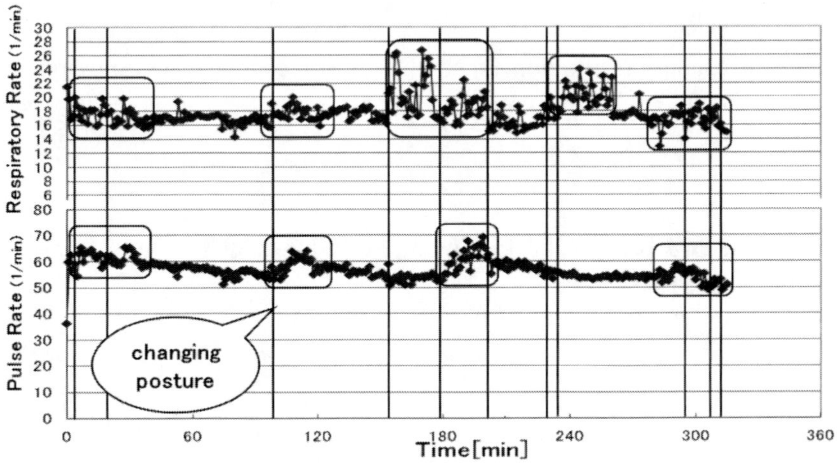

Figure 5.7. Transitions of changing posture added by solid lines on the graphs of rates of respiration and pulse shown in Figure 5.3.

The role of changing sleeping posture was then studied. With the transition of pulse rate as shown in Figure 5.3, significant numbers of pillars were described in Figure 5.6 as well as Figure 5.1. In Figure 5.6, the points at which changes in posture occurred are traced by thick vertical lines above and along the pulse rate transition. To consider the posture changes more clearly, the thick lines were overlaid vertically and lined up on two rate transitions as shown in Figure 5.7 by refining Figure 5.6.

In this latter figure, the pillars reaching to the level of zero were masked by interposing for ease of visibility. After all, it is the same as Figure 5.3. As a result, these lines were found to be related as follows:

(i)   The overlaid lines, i.e., changes of sleeping posture, are related to the occurrence of significant scale of fluctuation for the rates of respiration and pulse, as marked by quadrilaterals in Figure 5.7.

(ii)   This significant scale of fluctuation of respiration and pulse occurred at the overlaid lines, viz., change of sleeping posture, sometimes occurring simultaneously and sometimes not simultaneously.

(iii) At the time of posture change, rapid increases or decreases in pulse rate and/or respiration rate are observed.

Thus, A-BMWs introducing the change of postures occurred at the same time as significant variations or fluctuations in the rate of respiration and/or pulse, and especially respiration. In another words, change of sleeping posture is a trigger to increase or decrease the rates of respiration and/or pulse rapidly in a wide range.

5.4. Nature and Reasons for Change of Sleeping Posture in Unconscious State

Skeletal muscles – i.e., voluntary muscles other than those related to respiration and pulse – produce various body actions under the control of the somatic nervous system during the waking state. The present study affirmed that the change of sleeping posture occurred during sleep, i.e., the unconscious state, and found that such actions occurred not in a random order, but rather, as it were, in a physiological order: i.e., a physical desire to vary the rates of respiration and pulse to introduce remarkable variation or fluctuation. However, the autonomic nervous system is what controls rate transitions during sleep.

As a result, it cannot but be understood that an unconscious source such as the autonomic nervous system or reflexes gives order to skeletal muscles related to changing posture during sleep.

So what makes these sources give order? One interpretation – and it is just an interpretation – is that it may be considered a sort of 'crisis avoidance'. As we retain the same posture during sleep, certain areas of our body are placed under continuous pressure such that they begin to lack blood-flow and oxygen. Such a 'crisis' must be avoided by a change of sleeping posture, even if the cerebrum is not aware of it. Thus, the change of sleeping posture occurs to adjust body pressure distribution and to vary the circulation of blood and lymph fluid in the body.

As with this 'crisis avoidance' in the domain of the skeletal muscles, in the control of pulse rate by the autonomic nervous system, a similar crisis avoidance, or 'inconvenience avoidance', was seen in pulse rate transition, as described in the next section. One interpretation arising from this is that the autonomic nervous system and reflexes cooperate with each other to restore the mind and body during sleep.

6. HIGH-GRADE CONTROL FOR THE CARDIOVASCULAR SYSTEM

6.1. Reasons for, and Mechanism of Pulse Rate Control during Sleep

It was confirmed that as the human system was relaxed, respiration rate and pulse rate, particularly the latter, decreased. This gave rise to questions of why the rate did not remain low but rather increased and decreased periodically, what exactly happened at the lower and higher levels, and how these phenomena were affected by stimuli.

In order to investigate the mechanism of the rate control further, detailed transit of "instantaneous pulse rate" was studied, since minute pulse rate is only an average value which masks detailed behavior.

Figures 6.1(a) and 6.1(b) show examples of instantaneous pulse rate of three 5-minute portions, respectively, extracted from the data for the control and the music in Figure 4.5 [4]. As an initial result, as shown in Figure 6.1 (a), portions n_1 and n_3 at approximately middle level over the course of one night had fluctuations with a magnitude of less than approximately 10, while n_2 at higher level had fluctuations of 20 to 40.

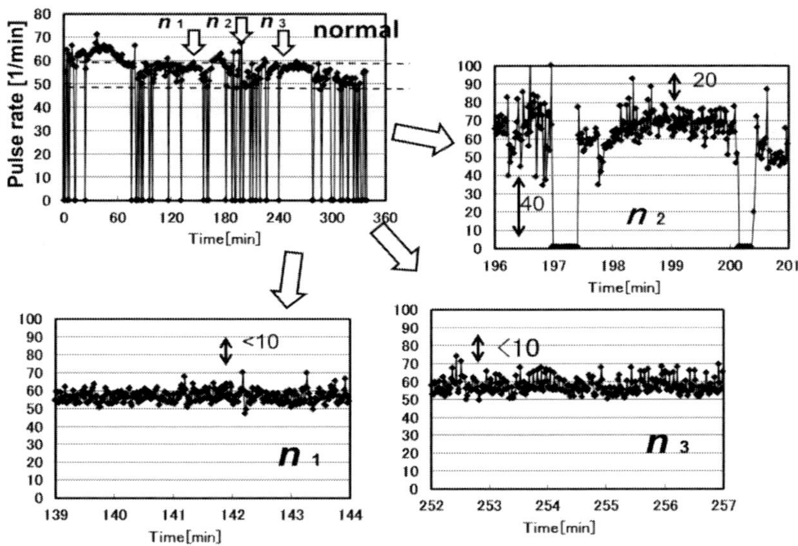

Figure 6.1. (a) Instantaneous pulse rates of three 5 minute portions.

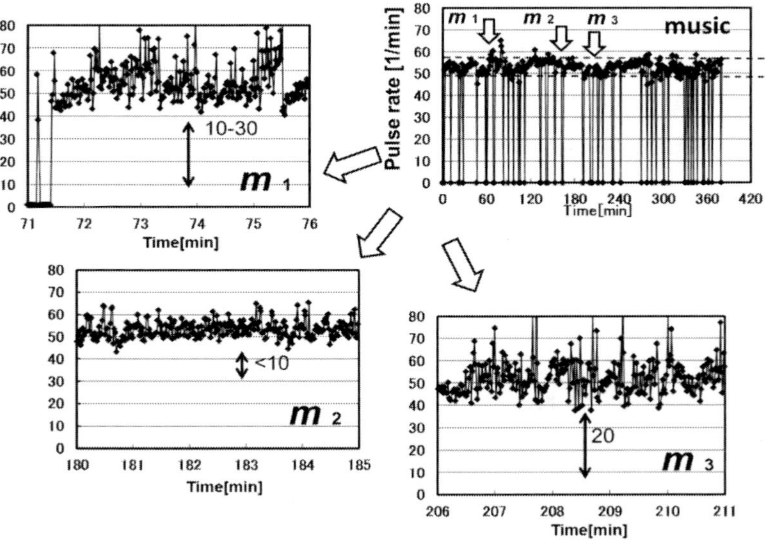

Figure 6.1. (b) Instantaneous pulse rates of three 5 minute portions.

In the second, in Figure 6.1 (b), portion m_2 at the middle level through one night had fluctuations with a magnitude of less than approximately 10. On the contrary, m_1 at the highest level of 60 bpm (in minute rate) had large magnitude fluctuation in the range 10 to 30, while m3 at the lowest level of 50 bpm (in minute rate) also showed large magnitude fluctuation of 20.

Though such investigation is still in progress, the fluctuation known from the instantaneous pulse rate implies that the autonomic nervous system determined approximately three pulse rate ranges as:

R_a: large magnitude in fluctuation of instantaneous pulse rate at larger minute pulse rate level;

R_b: less magnitude in fluctuation of instantaneous pulse rate at a certain range in minute pulse rate; and

R_c: large magnitude in fluctuation of instantaneous pulse rate at lower pulse rate level.

Such a specific minute pulse rate range R_b implies, as it were, an optimum range for a calm state of sleep. In this range, the heart beats with relative ease. However, minute pulse rate increases up to the range Ra, and then decreases down to the range R_c in alternating sequence, due to some unknown physiological reasons. Thus, once the minute pulse rate becomes larger up to the range Ra, the heart makes an effort to reduce the minute pulse rate by means of large magnitude of fluctuation in consecutive beats, i.e., instantaneous pulse rate, so as not to remain at a high rate or increase any further.

On the contrary, once the minute pulse rate enters the range R_c, the heart makes an effort to return to an appropriate rate in the range R_b by means of a large magnitude of fluctuation in instantaneous pulse so as not to remain at a lower rate or decrease any further.

Accordingly we suggest specific terms for the range R_b mentioned above as Minute Optimum Pulse Rate Range for Sleep (moPR-S). In addition, from this perspective, further study might suggest the magnitude range of fluctuation as 'Instantaneous Optimum Pulse Rate Range for Sleep' (ioPR-S).

6.2. Variation by Relaxation

As shown in Figure 4.5, minute pulse rate decreased. Then, as shown in Figure 6.1(a) (b), pulse rate range R_b shifted toward a lower level, i.e., moPR-S just decreased. The range moPR-S can be determined by approximately 51-60 for normal (i.e., non-stimulus) sleep as shown in Figure 6.1(a), and by approximately 48-57 for the stimulus, as shown in Figure 6.1(b), traced by dashed lines in the diagrams. Thus, it was found that music stimuli decreased the minute pulse rate and moPR-S shifted toward a lower level. However, it seemed that the stimuli did not induce large amplitude of fluctuation of instantaneous pulse rate in the ranges R_a and R_c.

CONCLUSION

Health in both body and mind is something we all want. However, we do not necessarily have a good understanding of what it is, or how to achieve it. This study has therefore sought to promote such understanding scientifically from a new viewpoint, which is that satisfaction in body and mind, health in body and mind, and good sleep can be connected by the autonomic nervous system. Autonomic nervous system activities can be observed to some extent in the waking state by vital signs, but are masked by large amounts of mental activity. The author therefore paid attention to phenomena which occur during sleep, since, in unconsciousness, mental activity takes a break. As a result, it was found that satisfaction can be measured physiologically through the study of unconscious behaviors.

Given that some of the issues of interest to researchers – food, lifestyle, athletics, dreams, sleep disorders, myocardial infarction during sleep, etc. – have not yet been fully explored, however, the present method may be able to contribute.

ACKNOWLEDGMENT

The author would like to acknowledge the subjects who participated in this study, as well as Carbon Technology Labo, Toyo Feather Industry Co. Ltd, Real Design Co. Ltd, Moss Japan Co. Ltd, M.I. Labo, Ohtake Root Kogyo Co. Ltd, and Nwic Co. Ltd for supplying materials for use in the experiment. The author would also like to acknowledge the Research Institute of Science and Technology for Science, Japan for NEXER project, 2009.

REFERENCES

[1]	Okawai, H., Ichisawa, S. and Numata, K. (2011). Detection of influence of stimuli or services on the physical condition and satisfaction with unconscious response reflecting activities of autonomic nervous system, N. A. Abu Osman et al. *(Eds.), BIOMED2011, IFMBE Proceedings, 35,* Kuala Lumpur, MALAYSIA, 20-23 June, 420-423.

[2]	Okawai, H., Kato, K. and Baya, D. (2012). Entrusting the reply of satisfaction or physical condition for services to unconscious responses reflecting activities of autonomic nervous system, 4th International *Conference on Applied Human Factors and Ergonomics, AHFE2012, San Francisco,* 21-25 July, 911-920.

[3]	Okawai, H., Yajima, T., Wada, J. and Takashima, M. (2014). Detection of Satisfaction for the Services by Body Motion Wave Revealing Unconscious Responses Reflecting Activities of Autonomic Nervous System, Ahram T, Karwowski W, Marek T (Eds.), *Proceedings of the 5th International Conference on Applied Human Factors and Ergonomics AHFE 2014, Krakow, Poland,* 19-23 July, 4297-4286.

[4]	Okawai, H., Yajima, T. and Mitsuru, Takashima. Physiological Detection of Satisfaction for Services by Body Motion Wave Revealing Unconscious Responses Reflecting Activities of Autonomic Nervous Systems. *3rd international conference on Serviceology (ICServ 2015),* 7pages, San Jose, CA, USA., July 7 - 9, 2015.

[5]	Kuno, H., Takashima, M. and Okawai, H. (2004). Measurement of Respiration, heart beat and body movement on a bed using dynamic air-pressure sensor, *IEEJ Trans. EIS.,* vol. *124,* No.4, 935-940 (in Japanese).

[6]	Okawai, H. and Kakegawa, H. Mitsuru Takashima; Body motion wave due to activities of autonomic nervous system applied to evaluation of bedding materials of carbon fiber. *The 12th IBRC (2015) Proceedings, Biophilia,* 2015(3), pp. 265-266. Fujisawa, Japan, Octber 22, 2015.

[7]	Hori, T. (2008). Sleep psychology, Kitaoji Shobou, Kyoto, Japan (in Japanese).

[8]	Kaniusas, E. (2012). *Sleep, Biomedical signals and Sensors 1,* Springer, 270-282.

[9] Okawai, H., Yajima, T. and Imamatsu, T. (2012). Transition of Rates of Respiration and Pulse, and Sleeping Posture During Night Detected by Body Motion Wave, IEEE international Conference on Biomedical Engineering and Sciences, Langkawi, *MALAYSIA*, 17-19 December, 129-133.

[10] Okawai, H., Yajima, T., Imamatsu, T. and Wada, J. (2013). Sophisticated Rate Control of Respiration and Pulse during Sleep Studied by Body Motion Wave. L. M. Roa Romero (eds.), *XIII Mediterranean Conference on Medical and Biological Engineering and Computing 2013, IFMBE Proceedings 41, MEDICON*, 2013, 25-28 September, Seville, Spain: 1895-1898.

INDEX

B

C

F

G

H

hair, 37, 78
hair cells, 37, 78
hardness, 140, 142
HBV, 74
head injury, 38, 81
healing, 135, 137, 140
healing music, 135, 137
health, x, 3, 31, 58, 69, 121, 122, 123, 124, 126, 129, 130, 154
health condition, 129, 130
health services, 31
heart disease, 31, 68, 123
heart failure, 6, 14, 15, 19, 34, 62, 67, 69, 70, 75, 88, 107, 108, 110, 112, 117
heart rate, viii, 5, 9, 12, 14, 15, 17, 27, 28, 29, 30, 31, 32, 33, 34, 41, 42, 45, 47, 60, 62, 63, 64, 65, 66, 67, 68, 69, 70, 71, 72, 73, 74, 75, 76, 77, 82, 83, 86, 87, 88, 90, 91, 92, 94, 95, 97, 98, 101, 102, 103, 104, 107, 109, 110, 111, 112, 114, 115, 117
heart transplantation, 17, 26
heme, 49, 100
hemodialysis, 14, 74, 82
hemorrhage, 106
hepatotoxicity, 75
herbicide, 108
history, 19, 113
homeostasis, 6
hormone(s), 37, 51, 98, 126, 130
hospice, 92
hospitalization, 95
house, 133, 143
housing, 123
human, 6, 7, 11, 18, 20, 25, 26, 49, 75, 76, 82, 94, 97, 105, 106, 125, 126, 127, 128, 130, 142, 151
human subjects, 6
hydroxyl, 20, 25
hygiene, 40
hyperemia, 6
hyperglycemia, 34, 65, 66, 86, 116
hypertension, 15, 19, 71, 87, 124

hyperthyroidism, 51, 103
hypoglycemia, 47, 94, 95, 103, 116
hypothalamus, vii, 2
hypothesis, viii, 28, 36, 41, 46, 48, 50, 92
hypothyroidism, 103
hypoxia, 38, 47, 49, 50, 63, 80, 94, 95, 96, 111, 116
hypoxia-inducible factor, 49

I

IL-13, 108
ileum, 25
immune activation, 108
immune response, 108, 116
immune system, 14, 71
immunohistochemistry, 8
immunosuppressive agent, 104
impairments, 32, 34, 54, 78
improvements, 7, 91, 116
impulses, 58
in vitro, 77, 78, 94
in vivo, 24, 77, 94
incidence, viii, ix, 28, 29, 36, 37, 39, 40, 43, 44, 45, 46, 49, 52, 55, 65, 69, 85, 98, 100, 109
India, 91, 101
individuals, x, 67, 76, 82, 114, 121
induction, 12, 38, 40, 60, 73, 82
industry, 41, 42, 43, 58, 59
infarcted myocardium, 7
infarction, 8, 10, 17, 18, 19, 20, 23, 24, 31, 62, 72, 75, 76, 88, 93, 98, 101, 107, 154
infection, ix, 29, 33, 38, 39, 40, 43, 44, 53, 55, 73, 110, 113, 117
inflammation, viii, ix, 8, 14, 16, 21, 23, 28, 35, 37, 49, 61, 63, 64, 66, 69, 70, 71, 74, 77, 92, 97, 99, 108, 113, 114
inflammatory arthritis, 103
inflammatory bowel disease, 70, 71
inflammatory disease, 45
ingestion, 63, 67, 110
inhibition, 21, 25, 35, 86, 102, 107
inhibitor, 43, 73, 86, 88, 107
initiation, 15, 68, 104

J

K

L

M

N

O

P

S

T

U

V

W

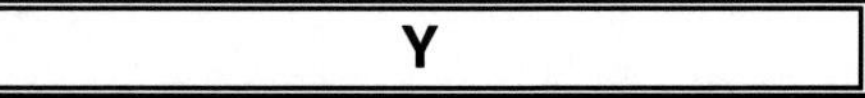
Y